2000

Error Reduction in Health Care

A Systems Approach to Improving Patient Safety

Patrice L. Spath, Editor

Jossey-Bass Publishers
San Francisco

Health Forum, Inc.
An American Hospital Association Company
CHICAGO

press

is a service mark of the American Hospital Association used under license by AHA Press.

Jossey-Bass books and products are available through most bookstores. To contact Jossey-Bass directly, call (888) 378-2537, fax to (800) 605-2665, or visit our website at www.josseybass.com.

Substantial discounts on bulk quantities of Jossey-Bass books are available to corporations, professional associations, and other organizations. For details and discount information, contact the special sales department at Jossey-Bass.

Manufactured in the United States of America on Lyons Falls Turin Book. This paper is acid-free and 100 percent totally chlorine-free.

Cover design by Laura Duggan

Library of Congress Cataloging-in-Publication Data

Error reduction in health care : a systems approach to improving
    patient safety / by Patrice L. Spath, editor.
        p.   cm.
    Includes index.
    ISBN 1-55648-271-X
    1. Health facilities—Risk management.   2. Medical errors—
Prevention.   I. Spath, Patrice.
RA971.38.E77   1999
362.1—dc21   99-37104
                                                                            CIP

FIRST EDITION
HB Printing   10 9 8 7 6 5 4 3 2 1

A wise person once said, "It is not the lofty sails but the unseen wind that moves the ship." This book is dedicated to Audrey Y. Kaufman, one of those unseen people who for more than 15 years helped to move the ship at AHA Press. Audrey's passion for excellence and unwavering belief in my editorial abilities made this book possible. I am proud to call her my friend.

Contents

List of Figures and Tables . . . . *vii*

About the Editor . . . . *xi*

About the Contributors . . . . *xiii*

Foreword . . . . *xxi*

Preface . . . . *xxv*

Acknowledgments. . . . . *xxxi*

CHAPTER 1

A Formula for Errors: Good People + Bad Systems
Susan McClanahan, RN, BSN,
Susan T. Goodwin, RN, MSN, and Frank Houser, MD

1

CHAPTER 2

Measuring Performance of High-Risk Processes
Karen Ferraco and Patrice L. Spath, BA, ART

17

CHAPTER 3

The Human Side of Medical Mistakes
Sven Ternov, MD

97

CHAPTER 4

Accident Investigation and Anticipatory Failure Analysis in Hospitals
Sanford E. Feldman, MD, FACS,
and Douglas W. Roblin, PhD

139

CHAPTER 5

Automating Root Cause Analysis
Robert J. Latino

155

CHAPTER 6

One Hospital's View of Software Facilitation
of Root Cause Analysis   165
Kenneth A. Hirsch, MD, PhD,
and Dennis T. Wallace, DABRM

CHAPTER 7

Proactively Error-Proofing Health Care Processes   179
Richard J. Croteau, MD, and Paul M. Schyve, MD

CHAPTER 8

Reducing Errors through Work System Improvements 199
Patrice L. Spath, BA, ART

CHAPTER 9

A Structured Teamwork System to Reduce
Clinical Errors   235
Daniel T. Risser, PhD, Robert Simon, MEd, EdD,
Matthew M. Rice, MD, JD, FACEP,
and Mary L. Salisbury, RN, MSN

Index   279

List of Figures and Tables

Figures

2-1   Activities That Must Be Regularly Evaluated in Health Care
Organizations Accredited by the Joint Commission 22

2-2   General Risk-Related Performance Measures 27

2-3   Examples of Performance Measures for Safety-Critical Tasks
in Major Patient Care Functions 33

2-4   Sample Hospital Incident Report 39

2-5   Definitions for Common Reportable Incidents 42

2-6   Sample Aggregate Incident Report for a Hospital 45

2-7   Occurrence Report. 46

2-8   Taxonomy of Medication Errors Recommended
by the National Coordinating Council for Medication Error
Reporting and Prevention, United States Pharmacopeia. 51

2-9   Patient Encounter Worksheet 70

2-10 Percentage of Children Overdue for Routine Immunizations
at Quarterly Intervals (July 1993 to April 1994) 71

2-11 Percentage of Patient Incidents That Did Not Result
in Discomfort, Infection, Pain, or Harm to the Patient 77

2-12 Control Chart Prototype 78

2-13 Clinical Profile 81

3-1   Typical Questions Asked during a Medical Accident
Investigation 112

3-2   Typical Medical Accident Trajectory. 113

3-3   Steps of the MTO Analysis. 120

3-4   Training and Support of the Team in MTO Analysis 121

4-1   Root Cause Analysis Results of the Death of a Patient
      Following Blood Transfusion (Case #1) 147

4-2   Retrospective Root Cause Analysis of Serious Disability
      Following Elective Arthroscopic Knee Surgery (Case #2). . . . 148

7-1   Levels of Analysis. 183

7-2   A Checklist for Proactive Risk-Reduction Activities 196

8-1   Work System Improvement Principles 204

8-2   Physicians' Order Sheet. 206

8-3   Patients' Role in Medication Usage. 213

8-4   Sample Family Education Guide for Infant Security 214

8-5   Strategies to Help Reduce the Risk
      of Restraint-Related Deaths. 217

8-6   Tips for Reducing Medication Errors
      in the Physician's Office. 221

9-1   Most Frequent Teamwork Errors 240

9-2   Care Resources Managed by the ED Core Team 243

9-3   The Interrelationships of the Five Team Dimensions 246

9-4   The Teamwork Check Cycle 251

9-5   Teamwork Failure Checklist 254

9-6   Individual Claim Assessment Process. 257

9-7   Example of Completed Teamwork Failure Checklist 261

9-8   Senior Leader Actions Necessary to Support
      Teamwork Implementation 269

9-9   Teamwork System Implementation. 271

Tables

2-1 Task Criticality Scoring System for the Process
of Warfarin Administration 32

2-2 ICD-9-CM Codes for Fetal Complications/Birth Injuries 67

2-3 Error Management Report for the High-Risk Activity
of Medication Usage. 75

3-1 Example of a Blank MTO Diagram 124

3-2 Taxonomy of Contributing Causes 127

3-3 Example of a Schematic Diagram from an MTO Analysis. . . . 129

6-1 Matrix to Use in Setting Priorities
for RCA Software Features 176

7-1 Probability of Success in a Process 185

9-1 Team Characteristics 245

9-2 Teamwork Behavior Matrix. 248

9-3 Potential Uses of Teamwork Failure Checklist Findings. 266

About the Editor

Patrice L. Spath, BA, ART, is a health care quality and information management specialist based in Forest Grove, Oregon. A much sought-after speaker, Ms. Spath has presented more than 350 educational programs on performance improvement, case management, patient safety improvement, clinical paths, and outcomes management. She has also authored several books, video programs, and journal articles on these subjects. For AHA Press she edited *Clinical Paths: Tools for Outcomes Management* (1994), *Medical Effectiveness and Outcomes* (1996), *Beyond Clinical Paths: Advanced Tools for Outcomes Management* (1997), and *Provider Report Cards* (1999). For Brown-Spath & Associates (www.brownspath. com), Ms. Spath has written several practical "how-to" books on health care quality and resource management topics.

Ms. Spath is a regular columnist for *Hospital Peer Review* and *Hospital Case Management,* newsletters published by American Health Consultants. She is also editor of *The Quality Resource,* the bimonthly newsletter of the Quality Management Section of the American Health Information Management Association. She served on a work group of the Agency for Health Care Policy and Research to assist in the development of a model for translating practice guidelines into review criteria, performance measures, and standards of quality. She was a member of the Clinical Guidelines Panel of the Veterans Health Administration and a member of the Clinical Path Work Group of the Association of Operating Room Nurses, Inc. In 1998 the American Health Information Management Association presented Ms. Spath with the Legacy Award for her significant contributions to the health information management profession through her writings and presentations.

About the Contributors

Richard J. Croteau, MD, is executive director for strategic initiatives at the Joint Commission on Accreditation of Healthcare Organizations. In this capacity he is responsible for oversight and coordination of a number of mission-critical activities, including ongoing accreditation process improvement initiatives and the Sentinel Event Policy. Earlier appointments at the Joint Commission include vice president for accreditation services, director of survey technology, director of the department of interpretation, associate director in the Hospital Accreditation Program, and hospital surveyor. Formerly, Dr. Croteau was chief of surgery and medical director at South County Hospital in Wakefield, Rhode Island. Prior to entering the health care field, he served as a rocket systems analyst for NASA's Lunar Module program, Project Apollo, White Sands, New Mexico, and as an instructor in computer programming at Brown University. He earned his bachelor's degree in aerospace engineering from Brown University and his medical degree from Boston University School of Medicine.

Sanford E. Feldman, MD, FACS, is a retired general surgeon whose research and practice interests have included medical quality and outcome assessment, impact of regulation on hospital staff monitoring, and error and system-fault in causing patient harm. He practiced surgery in San Francisco from 1946 to 1983 and was founding medical director of San Francisco Peer Review. He was medical director of the California Medicare PRO, CMRI, from 1984 to 1987, and assistant clinical professor of surgery at UCSF-Mt. Zion Medical Center in San Francisco. He received his MD from Stanford.

Karen Ferraco has been risk management consultant at ProNational Insurance Company in Okemos, Michigan, since 1995. She has specialized in risk management with an emphasis on professional and hospital liability for more than 18 years. She formerly served as a risk manage-ment supervisor for PHICO Insurance Company in Pennsylvania after providing risk management services for hospitals as a member of the field staff. In addition to her strengths in analyzing high-risk exposures, she practiced as a registered nurse for 10 years. Ms. Ferraco addresses medical and professional audiences on general, medical, and corporate liability issues. She is frequently involved in training and educational presentations for medical professionals and medical staff and hospital board members. She is affiliated with the American Society for Health-care Risk Management, the College of Healthcare Executives, the Asso-ciation of Operating Room Nurses, and the Medical Group Management Association. She graduated from the University of Pittsburgh with a BS degree in nursing, has her Associate in Risk Management designation, and is a Certified Healthcare Environmental Manager.

Susan T. Goodwin, RN, MSN, is director of quality management in the quality standards department for Columbia/HCA Healthcare Corporation in Nashville, Tennessee. She began her tenure with Columbia/HCA in 1985, and since then has served in various market and division-level positions prior to taking her current position in 1995. A graduate of the University of South Carolina, Ms. Goodwin's clinical experience includes nine years as a pediatric registered nurse. She received a master's degree in nursing administration in 1989 from Andrews University. She is a Certified Profes-sional of Healthcare Quality and a licensed risk manager in the state of Florida. She serves as a member of the clinical faculty of the Joint Com-mission on Accreditation of Healthcare Organizations. She is a contributor of articles and a public speaker on the topic of health care quality.

Kenneth A. Hirsch, MD, PhD, is a director of Medical Risk Manage-ment Associates, LLC, a risk management firm in San Diego, California (www.sentinel-event.com), which offers consulting, training, and com-puter software in medical risk management, sentinel event policy, and root cause analysis. He has worked in the area of risk management for the past seven years and currently serves on the editorial advisory boards of two sentinel event newsletters. He has had several articles and interviews in the medical risk management arena published. As a clinician, he has practiced in clinical psychology, psychiatry, and addic-tionology. He is currently head of inpatient psychiatry at a major med-ical center in San Diego.

Frank Houser, MD, is the chief medical director and senior vice president of quality at Columbia/HCA Physician Services in Nashville, responsible for developing corporate initiatives to ensure and improve the quality of services in Columbia/HCA facilities and for improving relationships with the 75,000 doctors on the active medical staff of Columbia/HCA hospitals and surgery centers. Dr. Houser entered the private practice of pediatrics in 1971 in Dalton, Georgia, moved to Atlanta, and started a medical group practice that provided all medical care to members of the PruCare HMO. For 11 years he was president of his group and medical director of the HMO. He was appointed public health director for the state of Georgia in 1991. He left state government in 1993, and after a brief stint at Emory he joined Columbia/HCA as president of the company's Georgia division. He is a graduate of Emory College and Emory Medical School.

Robert J. Latino is vice-president of strategic development for Reliability Center, Inc. (RCI), in Hopewell, Virginia. RCI is a reliability engineering firm specializing in improving equipment, process, and human reliability (see http://www.reliability.com). He has a special interest in the theory of human error as applied to failure analysis and is a practitioner of root cause analysis in the field with his clientele. He is also an educator and the author of RCI's *Root Cause Failure Analysis Methods* course, coauthor of RCI's *Failure Analysis/Problem Solving Methods for Field Personnel,* and coauthor of *Root Cause Analysis: Eliminating the Need to Do Work,* published by CRC Press in 1999. He has also published articles on failure analysis in numerous trade magazines and is a frequent speaker on that topic at trade conferences. He received his bachelor's degree in business administration and management from Virginia Commonwealth University.

Susan McClanahan, RN, BSN, is a director in the quality standards department of Columbia/HCA Healthcare Corporation in Nashville. She joined the company in 1995 and now works as a consultant to support Columbia/HCA's affiliated hospitals in the development of quality management programs, policies, and procedures. She is also actively involved in designing and monitoring systems to augment the hospitals' performance improvement efforts and supports their utilization review, management systems, credentialing, and other regulatory and accrediting activities. During her career, Ms. McClanahan has held various positions in acute care facilities. She is a registered nurse and has a BS in nursing from the University of Tennessee at Knoxville. She specialized in emergency department nursing for eight years before obtaining her certification as a paralegal and was claims investigator in risk management at Vanderbilt University Medical Center in 1990. She is a member of the American Society for Healthcare Risk Management and the Emergency Nurses Association.

Matthew M. Rice, MD, JD, FACEP, is a board-certified emergency physician with 20 years of emergency care experience, a fellow of the American College of Emergency Physicians, and an attorney. He is chief of the department of emergency medicine at Madigan Army Medical Center and program director for emergency medicine residency; assistant clinical professor at the Uniformed Services University of Health Sciences in Bethesda, Maryland; clinical assistant professor in medicine at the University of Washington in Seattle; and a board member on the National Patient Safety Foundation. In addition, Dr. Rice serves as a member of the incident review and risk management team for the medical center. Dr. Rice recently led the development and testing of the MedTeams Project teamwork training course and is a certified teamwork instructor.

Daniel T. Risser, PhD, is an experimental social psychologist with 20 years of research experience examining teams and organizations. He is a senior scientist in the Crew Performance Group at Dynamics Research Corporation in Andover, Massachusetts. He is a member of the American Society for Healthcare Risk Management (ASHRM), a member of the ASHRM Claim Data Gathering Task Force, and a former assistant professor of organizational behavior in a business school. Dr. Risser is currently the lead researcher examining clinical errors in a large, 10-hospital project (the MedTeams Project) designed to improve teamwork and reduce errors. He has also conducted research on the malpractice implications of medical teamwork failures. He previously conducted teamwork research on Army helicopter aircrews, conducted research on human design in weapon systems, and helped develop Human System Integration policy for weapon design for the Office of the Secretary of Defense.

Douglas W. Roblin, PhD, is senior research scientist with Kaiser Permanente's Georgia region. He joined Kaiser Permanente in 1988, working initially as a statistician and more recently as a health economist. Prior to this he was a statistician with the California Medicare PRO. His principal research interests are chronic disease epidemiology; neonatal and peri-natal care; primary care organization and practice variation; and methods for health risk, severity of illness, and quality of life measurement. He serves on advisory committees for the National Committee on Quality Assurance (Diabetes Quality Improvement Project) and the American Diabetes Association (Provider Recognition Program Steering Commit-tee) and is a member of the editorial advisory board for the Joint Com-mission on Quality Improvement. He has an MA from the University of Chicago and a PhD from the University of Michigan, both in anthropology.

Mary L. Salisbury, RN, MSN, is the director of the Institute for Quality Healthcare of Dynamics Research Corporation in Andover, Massachu-setts. Over the past few years Ms. Salisbury has been the coordinator of clinical research for emergency medicine at Rhode Island Hospital and in this role has been a principal participant in the development of the MedTeams Project teamwork system and is a certified teamwork instructor. She has had 30 years in critical care/emergency care nursing and has worked as a staff nurse, assistant clinical manager, and clinical manager of a Level I trauma center. She also served as senior human resource representative in negotiations with unions and clinical liaison to risk management for incidents and claims review.

Paul M. Schyve, MD, is the senior vice president of the Joint Com-mission on Accreditation of Healthcare Organizations. From 1989 until 1993 he was vice president for research and standards and before that director of standards at the Joint Commission. Prior to joining the Joint Commission, he was the clinical director of the State of Illinois Depart-ment of Mental Health and Developmental Disabilities. He received an undergraduate degree from the University of Rochester, where he was elected to Phi Beta Kappa. He completed his medical education and residency in psychiatry at the University of Rochester and has subse-quently held a variety of professional and academic appointments in the areas of mental health and hospital administration, including serv-ing as director of the Illinois State Psychiatric Institute and clinical associate professor of psychiatry at the University of Chicago. Dr. Schyve is certified in psychiatry by the American Board of Psychiatry and Neurology and is a fellow of the American Psychiatric Association. He has published in the areas of psychiatric treatment and research, quality assurance, continuous quality improvement, health care accreditation, and health care ethics.

Robert Simon, MEd, EdD, is the chief scientist and manager of the Crew Performance Group at Dynamics Research Corporation in Andover, Massachusetts, and the principal investigator and program manager of the MedTeams Project, which has developed and validated a teamwork training and implementation system for the emergency departments of hospitals (see http://teams.drc.com). Dr. Simon has also conducted teamwork research on Army helicopter crews and Air Force combat crews and used those research results to establish successful teamwork training courses to improve mission effectiveness and flight safety. He has also conducted aviation human factors research to improve equipment design. He trained in behavioral research and evaluation at the University of Massachusetts and has had 20 years of research experience in curriculum development, teamwork training, and human factors. He is a certified human factors professional (CPE) and a member of the Human Factors and Ergonomics Society.

Sven Ternov, MD, a physician specializing in general medicine, is an inspector for the Swedish Board of Health and Welfare at the regional unit in Malmoe. Since 1991 he has served as the medical supervisor of numerous accident investigations in Swedish health care facilities. In this role he has developed a rigorous medical accident analysis process based on methods used by the nuclear power industry. He has taught classes on his method for the Swedish and Danish Board of Health and advised health care providers on quality assurance issues, especially in regard to preventive measures and how to improve the efficacy and safety of processes. Also trained as a lead auditor on the ISO 9000 quality system standard, Dr. Ternov has performed a number of audits for clinical services in health care. For the past three years he has been engaged in research on design principles for the human-machine (system) interface at the Lund Institute of Technology, University of Lund, Sweden. His interests lie in designing safe and reliable interfaces to optimize the problem-solving environment for a problem solver in "the sharp end" of a system. He is also involved in validating a method (DEB analysis) for prospective reliability analysis of health care processes. He has published extensively in Sweden and lectured throughout Europe on systems for improving patient safety in health care.

Dennis T. Wallace, DABRM, is a director of Medical Risk Management Associates, LLC, a risk management firm in San Diego (www.sentinel-event.com), which offers consulting, training, and computer software in medical risk management, sentinel event policy, and root cause analysis. He currently serves on the editorial advisory board of a sentinel event newsletter and has published in the area of medical risk management. He has worked in the medical risk management arena for nine years and currently is the risk manager of a major medical center in San Diego.

Foreword

O ne would never guess from reading the chapters in this volume how new the error prevention movement in health care is. Five years ago, no one would have thought to publish such a book. Nor would many have read it. After all, it was just in 1995 that a series of tragic medical errors brought the issue to the public's and the profession's attention in a compelling way. That increasing awareness led, just a year later in October 1996, to the first Annenberg Conference on Examining Errors in Health Care, which brought together for the first time people from many different disciplines to talk and learn about a subject that was previously taboo and on which many had worked in isolation. At that meeting, too, leaders from medicine, nursing, pharmacology, and hospitals, as well as accreditors and regulators, for the first time acknowledged the need to improve patient safety and, more important, pledged to do it.

Since then, the idea that human errors are caused by bad systems, not bad people, has been accepted as a given. We ask now how to improve our systems, not how to catch "bad apples." We are creating nonpunitive environments for reporting errors. We are redesigning our systems. What a sea change!

Well, not quite. This patient safety movement, while clearly viable, is still in its infancy. Most hospitals have not stopped punishing for errors; most have not begun to redesign their systems; most regulatory bodies still search for villains and punish those who get caught. We have much to learn about how to create a culture of safety that even remotely compares to that which exists in aviation, nuclear power, and other hazardous industries.

The error numbers are staggering: serious medication errors alone occur in the case of 5 to 10 percent of patients admitted to hospitals, and lesser errors occur 10 times as often. And medication errors, the most studied and among the most visible of medical errors, are but a fraction of the total. When studies are limited to high-risk areas such as emergency rooms and intensive care units, rates of preventable injury are higher still.

The reasons are not obscure. The delivery of health care is incredibly complex. Managing sophisticated technology and powerful, dangerous drugs alone poses a daunting challenge. Add our unique combination of diverse patients, multiple processes, and various professional disciplines, loosely organized with unclear lines of authority and major communication barriers, and you have, to put it politely, a human factors engineering design nightmare. We have much to do!

Yet much has been accomplished in a very short time. The formation of the National Patient Safety Foundation by the American Medical Association has brought the many stakeholders to the table for productive dialogue and positive action. The Joint Commission on the Accreditation of Healthcare Organizations has implemented a nonpunitive sentinel events reporting system, and, under the leadership of the Veterans Health Administration, a public-private partnership has been created that brings together key government agencies and health care groups to advance the cause of patient safety.

Meanwhile, in several hundred hospitals, quality improvement teams have begun to address the problem of error prevention. Many have focused on medication safety. They have implemented a variety of process changes, such as revamping their chemotherapy programs, instituting protocols for hazardous drugs, and standardizing prescribing practices. Major systems changes, such as automated drug dispensing and computerized physician ordering systems, have appeared and hold great promise for substantially reducing serious errors. A number of hospitals have experimented with nonpunitive reporting programs for medication errors. The results in some individual nursing units have sometimes been phenomenal: 10-, 15-, 20-fold increases in the number of medication errors reported!

So there is activity, and there is progress, but it is frustratingly slow. Health care is undergoing a profound culture change in which all workers, from the CEO to the newest orderly, learn to feel personal responsibility for patient safety, and where discovering and reporting errors is rewarded, not punished. It is counterintuitive and flies in the face of much that we teach and have been taught. But systems theory is solidly based in science. Even more important, it works, and therefore it will prevail. It's just not easy.

The contributions in this book will advance that process. The intellectual basis for the systems approach—the concept of latent errors, situational factors, and defective barriers as the underlying causes of active errors—is clearly described by several authors. The application of human factors principles to design of tasks, processes, and systems is extensive, clearly presented, and illustrated by real-life examples that clinicians or patients can readily understand and relate to. The difficult area of error measurement is addressed as well in the context of performance measurement, also with extensive examples of application to clinical situations. While the discussion of automating root cause analysis is inconclusive, defining criteria advances the process.

Finally, two subjects in this book will be new to many readers and are, I think, evidence of the maturing of our approach to error prevention: prospective systems analysis and team training. Much has been made in the past about the importance of investigating accidents after they happen to uncover the underlying latent errors and systems failures. Few would question the necessity to learn from our mistakes. Yet many accidents, particularly so-called sentinel events, may well be "outliers" that give mixed or unclear messages about the status of the systems. Further, hindsight bias and lingering concerns about being blamed degrade the value of many of these investigations.

On the other hand, prospective evaluation of potentially hazardous situations—asking the "what if" question—suffers from neither of these limitations. It is not difficult for front-line workers to identify the hazardous situations—accidents waiting to happen—and they often welcome the opportunity to brainstorm about them and participate in efforts to redesign for safety. Two chapters offer valuable perspectives on prospective evaluation and provide tools for those who wish to explore this frontier more fully.

Team training is also a welcome addition—an idea whose time is long overdue. While many pay homage to the concept, efforts in the past to operationalize team training in a meaningful way, particularly in hazardous environments, have been haphazard at best. No single chapter can tell you all you need to know about the subject, but what we have here is a good introduction, and it is buttressed by a unique description of how to analyze and correct team malfunctions that lead to errors.

This volume, then, breaks new ground in important ways. It moves beyond the "why" to the "how," offering a wealth of innovative, valuable, and, most of all, useful ideas on how to create a safe environment for patient care. The "movement" is in good hands.

Lucian L. Leape, MD
Harvard School of Public Health

Preface

W hile millions of Americans receive medical care every day in one of the world's safest health care systems, high-profile cases have brought medical errors to the public's attention. In December 1995, a seven-year-old Florida boy died after receiving adrenaline instead of lidocaine during anesthesia for ear surgery. In 1997, the death of a Houston newborn made the cover of *The New York Times Magazine* after it was discovered that he had received an injection of the heart drug digoxin at 10 times the appropriate dose.

The public's perception of how often medical errors occur is alarmingly high. A 1997 Louis Harris & Associates poll of more than 1,500 Americans conducted for the National Patient Safety Foundation revealed that a large percentage of respondents (42 percent) felt that they or a close friend or relative had experienced a medical mistake. Several national organizations, including the Joint Commission, the Anesthesia Patient Safety Foundation, the Institute for Safe Medication Practices, the National Patient Safety Foundation, the Veterans Health Administration, and others are encouraging health care organizations to take steps to prevent errors, reduce error occurrence, and mitigate the effects of errors.

Error reduction in health care is what this book is all about. In the pages that follow you'll learn about reactive and proactive methods of patient safety improvement. When undesirable accidents occur, health care organizations should analyze the incident to find root causes and fix underlying system problems to prevent recurrence of a similar event (reactive). In addition, high-risk processes must be monitored and analyzed to identify where additional safeguards are needed to reduce the likelihood of an undesirable event (proactive).

In chapter 1, McClanahan, Goodwin, and Houser provide an overview of the issues surrounding health care accidents. Using a real-life case study, the authors describe how our system of care actually fosters mistakes. And although errors are often attributed to the action of an individual, there is usually a set of external forces and preceding events that lead up to the error. Quality experts agree that the most common cause of performance problems is the system itself, not the individuals functioning within the system. While a human error may have occurred, the root cause is likely to be found in the design of the system that permitted such an error to be made. The professionals that work together to provide patient care do not function in isolation. The activities of caregivers are influenced by multiple factors, including personal characteristics, attitudes, and qualifications; the composition of teams, organizational culture, and climate; physical resources; and the condition of the patient. These factors affect performance as well as influence decision making, task prioritization, and conflict resolution.

Accident investigators have found that most disasters in complex organizations had long incubation periods characterized by a number of discrete events signaling danger that were often overlooked or misinterpreted during the incubation period. This observation has important implications for health care organizations. Patient safety can be enhanced with the introduction of measures that continually evaluate risk-prone processes. By monitoring the performance of these processes, health care professionals can detect impending problems before an undesirable event occurs. Included in chapter 2 is advice on how to select the important tasks that should be regularly evaluated. The authors offer a scoring matrix that can be used to identify safety-critical patient care activities. More than 100 performance measures for high-risk processes, such as medication administration, restraint, and patient assessment, are included in this chapter. When danger signals become evident, changes in the process can be introduced to prevent a disaster from occurring.

The study of human errors in medicine is a relatively new field with researchers still trying to define the boundaries, terminology, and taxonomy. Nevertheless, a basic understanding of the kinds of errors health care professionals make can help us design better systems. In chapter 3 Ternov draws from previous work in the cognitive sciences and analyses of human performance to provide an in-depth review of the causes of medical mistakes. Ternov, principal investigator of medical accidents for the Board of Health and Welfare in Sweden, describes several medical accidents and near-miss events and provides insight into why they occurred and ways to keep them from recurring. He also details a unique method used in Sweden to proactively study high-risk health care processes so that preventive measures can be taken before a significant adverse event occurs.

Feldman has been studying the causes of sentinel events since the early 1960s. In chapter 4, he and Roblin of Kaiser Permanente show how the private industry model of root cause analysis can be applied to untoward patient care events to find the underlying causes. You'll learn how to identify the root causes of adverse events and fix the latent system problems that contribute to medical accidents. For a number of years complex technical industries have used computerized root cause analysis tools to investigate accidents and select root causes. Many people in health care are wondering if these tools are applicable to patient care processes. Chapters 5 and 6 address the role of computerized accident analysis tools and what one health care provider discovered when examining various RCA software choices.

If health care organizations are to improve patient safety, patient care processes must be designed to be more resistant to error occurrence and more accommodating of its consequences. It is not enough to wait for an accident to happen and then start improving patient care tasks. Better system reliability cannot be achieved by acting only on what is learned from yesterday's mistakes—proactive patient safety initiatives should be used to keep ahead of the accidents. If errors cannot be completely eliminated, then clinicians must learn how to quickly recognize the mistake and take appropriate actions to mitigate the consequences. In chapters 7 and 8 readers learn how to reduce the incidence of errors in many high-risk processes and what must be done to ensure that caregivers rapidly respond should a mistake occur. The authors also detail the accident-prevention recommendations of national organizations involved in tracking errors and adverse events in health care.

The aviation industry has discovered that faulty teamwork among crew members is a frequent causal factor in airline accidents. Many scientists involved in improving airline crew performance are now applying the same concepts to health care teams. By adopting structured teamwork improvement strategies, caregivers are finding that medical accidents can be prevented. Tactics for enhancing teamwork and communication among health care professionals are included in chapter 9. This groundbreaking work, used by teams in hospital emergency departments, is likely to result in significant patient care improvements.

In this chapter readers will find a checklist that can be used to identify the teamwork and communication problems that lead to an adverse patient event as well as a teamwork improvement action plan.

Medical accidents, near-miss situations, and recommendations for preventing these events are not new topics. For example, in 1886 Dr. Frank Hamilton wrote that "a few years ago a strong, healthy women died in the dentist's chair in New York City while under the influence of nitrous oxide."[1] Hamilton then goes on to describe how future events of this sort might be prevented, saying, "The danger to life would no doubt in these cases be diminished if the patient were in the recumbent position. Recent experiments and observations seem to have shown that the admixture of oxygen gas with the nitrous oxide in certain proportions averts the danger of asphyxia, while it does not diminish the anesthesia." In 1915 Gordon Christine, MD, wrote about problems related to ownership of patient records. According to Christine, "there is a widespread notion among nurses that bedside clinical records of a patient are the property of the attending nurse, and that they can therefore be rightfully removed by her from the home of the patient at the conclusion of her services."[2] Christine relates an incident in which the nurse took a patient's chart and refused to return it even though the continuity of care was being compromised. In two other instances Christine notes that records were removed "because the nurses wished to cover up some of their mistakes."

Today, media attention and growing concerns about the costs associated with medical mistakes have caused error reduction in health care to become a national imperative. How will the health care industry deal with this challenge? The old ways simply won't suffice—the issues are too complex. For example, we can't tackle the problem of medication errors by simply disciplining the people who make the mistakes. And we can't address patient safety improvement by looking for quick fixes. Instead, we need to adopt the error management principles and techniques that have reduced accidents in other complex, high-risk industries. Through a better understanding of the error environment, these industries have been able to design systems that promote error prevention as well as error recovery. Health care professionals must learn what causes mistakes to occur and then redesign processes to prevent or reduce error occurrence. Because it is impossible to eliminate all errors or perfectly design all systems, patient care processes should also be able to catch errors before they reach the patient.

Maintaining an organizational culture of safety and reliability is crucial to error reduction in health care. Organization leaders must realize the need for a comprehensive patient safety initiative and support the adoption of practices that enable physicians, managers, and staff to do their jobs without causing patient harm.

Patrice L. Spath, BA, ART
Health Care Quality Specialist
Forest Grove, Oregon

References

1. F. H. Hamilton. *The Principles and Practice of Surgery* (New York: William Wood & Company, 1886), p. 946.

2. G. M. Christine. "The Relation of the Nurse to the Ownership of Clinical Records," *The Trained Nurse and Hospital Review* 60, no. 1 (July 1915): 22–23.

Acknowledgments

The authors have many people to thank for their help in creating the concepts and techniques discussed in this book. First and foremost we must thank those practitioners who were willing to candidly describe mistakes they'd made and the factors surrounding these situations. Next, we thank those in industries outside of health care that have developed and refined the many accident investigation and error management methods that we are now beginning to use in health care organizations. Last, and most important, we wish to acknowledge the patients who experienced the adverse events described in these chapters. Although any medical accident is deplorable, the lives of future patients will be saved by what we are learning from examining these incidents.

1

A Formula for Errors:
Good People + Bad Systems

Susan McClanahan, RN, BSN
Susan T. Goodwin, RN, MSN
Frank Houser, MD

Mr. Murphy slipped on a wet floor in the locker room of the club-
house at his favorite golf course. He fell heavily on his right hip and
was in pain when he arrived by ambulance at the hospital's emergency department (ED). While Murphy was being examined, Mr.
Jenkins was also being admitted to the ED. Jenkins was a resident
of a local long-term care facility and he had also fallen on his right
side that morning.

In addition to caring for Murphy and Jenkins, the ED staff were
very busy with other patients. As was typical when the department
was crowded, the admissions registrar was behind in making
patient identification (ID) bands. The equipment used to make the
bands was old, and the process took some time. The registrar's time
was also occupied by other duties. As usually happened in this situation, the caregivers still ordered needed diagnostic tests and provided other patient care, simply remembering to verbally verify
patients' identity rather than checking ID bands. Orders for right hip
x-rays for both Murphy and Jenkins were entered into the computer
by the nursing staff.

Murphy was transported to the x-ray department first. According
to the usual practice, no documentation accompanied him. A requisition for an x-ray of the right hip was printed out in the radiology
department. The x-ray technician took the requisition from the
printer and, noting that it was for a right hip x-ray, verbally confirmed
with Murphy that he was there for this exam. The technician did not

1

check Murphy for an ID band since patients frequently arrived from the ED without a band in place, and he did not ask the patient his name. Unfortunately, the x-ray requisition was for Jenkins and it was Jenkins' name that was placed on Murphy's x-rays.

While x-rays were being taken of Murphy's hip, Jenkins was transported to the radiology department. A technician who had just come back from her lunch break took the Murphy requisition from the department's printer and confirmed with the transporter that the patient on the stretcher was there for a right hip x-ray. (Jenkins was not coherent enough to speak for himself.) She proceeded to perform the diagnostic study. The technician did not know that there was another patient in the department for the same study, and she assumed she had the right requisition for the right patient (essentially repeating the error of the first technician). Murphy's name was then placed on Jenkins' x-rays.

After both patients were transported back to the ED, the radiologist called the ED to report that the x-rays labeled with Murphy's name indicated a fracture. The x-rays labeled with Jenkins' name were negative for a fracture. Because metabolic diagnostic studies done on Jenkins indicated other medical problems, he was admitted to the hospital. Murphy was also admitted with a diagnosis of "fractured right hip." The radiologist had not been given any clinical information related to either patient. If he had, he may have noted that one of Murphy's diagnoses was obesity and his x-rays showed very little soft tissue. Jenkins, moreover, was very frail and thin and his x-rays showed a large amount of soft tissue.

Having been diagnosed with a fractured hip, Murphy was referred to an orthopedist. The orthopedist employed a physician assistant (PA) who performed a preoperative history and physical examinations, noting in the medical record that there was shortening and internal rotation of the right leg. The orthopedic surgeon did not personally confirm these findings prior to authenticating the history and physical examination, even though he had had to admonish the PA in the past for doing less-than-thorough exams. The orthopedic surgeon had not communicated the performance issues related to the PA to anyone at the hospital. Likewise, the hospital's quality management department did not collect or report performance measurement data for any allied health practitioners.

Surgery for Murphy was scheduled for the next day. Meanwhile, Jenkins continued to complain of severe pain in his right hip and refused to bear weight on that side. A repeat x-ray of his right hip was ordered and done late that evening. The radiologist read the x-ray the next morning and a fracture was noted. Although the staff recognized the discrepancy in diagnoses between the first and second x-rays, no immediate investigation of the reason for this was done. The case was merely flagged for retrospective peer review.

At the time of Murphy's scheduled surgery, the radiology department transported his x-rays to the surgical suite. However, the x-rays were not posted on the viewbox. Therefore, the discrepancy between the patient's physique and the soft tissue evident in the x-rays was not detected. Surgery proceeded until after the incision was made and the surgeon found no fracture. While waiting for the patient to recover from anesthesia, the surgeon made a quick call to the hospital risk manager to discuss how he should deliver the news of the unnecessary surgery to Murphy and his family.[1]

How often do incidents involving patient harm actually occur? A 1993 report compiled by the Harvard Malpractice Study indicated that approximately 1 million potentially preventable medical errors result in about 120,000 deaths each year.[2] In a more recent study, researchers examined 1,047 hospital records and discovered that 185 (17.7 percent) of the patients had at least one serious adverse event.[3] Although at first glance these numbers may appear high, medical errors resulting in adverse patient outcomes occur in only a very small percent of patient care encounters. The likelihood of an unnecessary surgery such as the one described in this introductory scenario is remote.

What is very common are the circumstances surrounding unnecessary surgery incidents. Emergency department staff are frequently busy caring for patients. Aged equipment routinely frustrates people's good intentions of doing their job well. Staff don't always follow procedures exactly as they are written. Conflicting diagnostic test findings may not get investigated right away. Clinicians periodically have insufficient information about the patients under their care. And yet patients are rarely harmed. Why? Because these circumstances may not cause a human error or, if an error does happen, it is detected and resolved before patient injury occurs. Mr. Murphy was the unlucky victim of less-than-ideal circumstances that led to a series of human errors that were not caught and corrected. Just as James Reason observed, the greatest risk of accident in a complex system such as health care is "not so much from the breakdown of a major component or from isolated operator errors, as from the insidious accumulation of delayed human errors."[4]

Recent high-profile cases have brought medical errors to the public's attention, and patient safety has become a growing concern for the public, policymakers, and all those who are involved in the delivery of health care services.[5-12] This chapter provides a general overview of the causes of medical mistakes and what can be done to eliminate or reduce the occurrence of such errors. Although the standard of medical practice is perfection (error-free patient care), most health care professionals recognize that mistakes are inevitable.[13] In this book, readers will discover how to examine medical mistakes and learn from them. This chapter is designed to set the stage for this learning by providing an overview of error management theories and techniques.

WHY MISTAKES OCCUR

Mistakes are unintended human acts (either of omission or commission) or an act that does not achieve its intended goal. No one likes to make mistakes, but everyone is quick to point them out. In the minds of society and medical professionals alike, mistakes are unacceptable. Why are health care professionals so quick to find fault and place blame? Psychologists call it "the illusion of free will." "People, especially in Western cultures, place great value in the belief that they are free agents, the captains of their own fate."[14] Because people are seen as free agents, their actions are viewed as voluntary and within their control. Therefore medical mistakes have traditionally been blamed on clinicians who were careless, incompetent, or thoughtless.

However, since human action is always limited by local circumstances, free will is an illusion, not a certainty.[15] Investigations of incidents such as the Three Mile Island and the Challenger disasters indicate that "accidents are generally the outcome of a chain of events set in motion by faulty system design that either induces errors or makes them difficult to detect."[16] Murphy's unnecessary surgery event illustrates the relationship between human errors and faulty systems. Several erroneous decisions and actions were made that had an immediate impact on the chain of events. These types of errors, known as active errors, are often conspicuous and recognized as slips, mistakes, and violations of rules or accepted standards of practice. Active errors are usually committed by the persons who appeared to be in control of the system at the time the accident evolved. Examples of active errors that occurred in the unnecessary surgery event included the following:

- Admissions registrar did not make patient ID bands in a timely manner.
- ED physicians and nursing staff proceeded with patient care activities even though patients did not have ID bands.
- X-ray technicians did not verbally verify patient names to match x-ray requisitions with the right patient.
- Staff did not immediately question the diagnostic discrepancy between Mr. Jenkins' first x-ray and his second x-ray.
- The orthopedic surgeon did not confirm the physical findings reported by the PA who performed Murphy's preoperative examination.
- Operating room staff did not ensure that Murphy's x-rays were posted on the viewbox in the operating room prior to the start of the procedure.

Through their errors, these "frontline operators" created the local immediate conditions that allowed the latent faults in the system to become manifest. Latent system faults are erroneous decisions and actions, often made by administration, that have a delayed impact on the function of the system.[17] Many times these latent system faults are only recognized after an incident occurs. Some of the system faults that created the background conditions that made the occurrence of an unnecessary surgery possible are listed below:

- Staffing for the admissions registration area was not adequate for the volume of patients experienced during the busier times in the ED. There was no contingency plan to increase staffing during these times. Instead, the staff prioritized their workload and improperly prioritized production of ID bands as a task that could wait. There were no policies and procedures set forth to guide staff more properly in what to do in a busy situation.

- The equipment used to produce ID bands was outdated and inefficient, which did not create problems during slow times but did when the volume of patients increased. This situation created the background condition for an accident.
- The staff had become desensitized to working during busier times with patients who did not have an ID band. They learned to cope by verifying a patient's identity verbally, and this practice became acceptable over time. This unwritten alternative procedure relied on the staff's remembering to ask, and it bypassed a safety-critical step in patient care delivery. It also further defied safety measures in the case of Mr. Jenkins, who was not able to verbally confirm his identity.
- There was a lack of communication of important information. Patient identification was not appropriately communicated between departments and caregivers. The radiologist did not receive any clinical information other than "rule out hip fracture" on the x-ray requisition forms. The x-rays were not posted in the surgery suite as a means of communicating significant patient information to the surgeon.
- The quality management activities of the hospital did not cover an entire category of care providers. There was no performance measurement data for allied health practitioners, including the PA. Traditionally, the quality management activities of the hospital most frequently resulted in peer review letters of sanction, and fear of this had prevented the orthopedic surgeon from communicating performance information about the PA for whom he was responsible. The surgeon also did not provide adequate supervision of the PA.

As shown by the accident scenario, adverse patient incidents rarely result from a single mistake. System safeguards and the abilities of caregivers to identify and correct errors before an accident occurs make single-error accidents highly unlikely. Rather, accidents typically result from a combination of latent failures, active errors, and breach of defenses.[18] The evidence from a large number of accident inquiries indicates that bad events are more often the result of error-prone situations and error-prone activities than they are of error-prone people.[19]

The balance of scientific opinion clearly favors system improvements rather than individual discipline as the desired error management approach for the following reasons:[20]

- Human fallibility can be moderated up to a point, but it can never be eliminated entirely. It is a fixed part of the human condition partly because, in many contexts, it serves a useful function (for example, trial-and-error learning in knowledge-based situations).
- Different types of errors have different psychological mechanisms, occur in different parts of the organization, and require different methods of management.
- Safety-critical errors happen at all levels of the system; they are not just committed by those directly involved in patient care.
- Measures that involve sanctions, threats, fear, appeals, and the like have only a very limited effectiveness, and in many cases they can harm morale, self-respect, and a sense of justice.
- Errors are a product of a chain of causes in which the precipitating psychological factors—momentary inattention, misjudgment, forgetfulness, preoccupation—are often the last and least manageable links in the chain.

Health care professionals have come to realize that individuals are not the primary cause of occasional sporadic accidents. They can, in fact, be the active agents of patient safety by identifying and eliminating those factors that undermine people's ability to do their jobs successfully.[21] In the next section of this chapter readers are introduced to the science of human factors analysis and what health care organizations can learn from the error-reduction efforts in other complex industries.

HOW TO ERROR-PROOF PROCESSES

Systems that rely on error-free human performance are destined to fail. Traditionally, however, individuals have been expected to not make errors. The time has come for health care professionals to admit that mistakes happen and aim improvement activities at the underlying system faults rather than at the people who make mistakes. For example, if a nurse gives the wrong medication to a patient, typically two things occur. First, an occurrence report is completed and sent to the nurse's department manager and risk management. Next, the nurse is "counseled" by management to pay closer attention next time. She is possibly told to read educational materials on the type of medication that was given in error. She may be warned that a second incident will result in a letter of reprimand being placed in her personnel file. However, these individual-focused actions won't fix the latent system failures that continue to smolder behind the scenes and will again manifest themselves when another medication error is made by a different nurse.

The discipline of human factors engineering (HFE) has been dealing with the causes and effects of human error since the 1940s. Originally applied to the design of military aircraft cockpits, HFE has since been effectively applied to the problem of human error in nuclear power plants, NASA spacecraft, and computer software.[22] The science of HFE has more recently been applied to health care systems to identify the causes of significant errors and develop ways to eliminate or ameliorate them.

Anesthesiologists were one of the first groups to recognize the importance of system redesign as an error reduction strategy.[23] The Anesthesia Patient Safety Foundation (APSF) was formed by the American Society of Anesthesiologists in 1984 with the goal of ensuring that no patient is harmed by the effects of anesthesia. To achieve this goal, the APSF participates in several initiatives, including the following:

- Sharing the results of investigations into anesthesia-related adverse events to provide a better understanding of how system improvements can prevent anesthetic injuries[24-27]
- Developing and making available anesthesia simulators directed at crisis management as well as teaching basic anesthesia skills[28]
- Evaluating the effect of fatigue on acuity, monitoring of intraoperative carbon monoxide levels, cerebral ischemia thresholds, and factors affecting intraoperative vigilance[29-31]

The American Society of Anesthesiologists was also one of the first medical professional groups to develop and disseminate clinical practice guidelines. This initiative in combination with system improvements has appeared to significantly reduce anesthesia-related mortality.[32]

By adopting the error-reduction strategies that have been successfully applied in other industries, many health care delivery systems can be redesigned to significantly lessen the likelihood of errors. Some of the tactics that have been summarized in health care literature by Leape and others are listed below:[33-36]

- *Reduce reliance on memory.* Work should be designed to minimize the need for human tasks that are known to be particularly fallible, such as short-term memory and vigilance (prolonged attention). Checklists, protocols, and computerized decision aids are examples of tools that could be incorporated into health care processes.
- *Improve information access.* Creative ways must be developed for making information more readily available; for example, displaying information where it is needed, when it is needed, and in a form that permits easy access by those who need it.
- *Error-proof processes.* Where possible, critical tasks should be structured so that errors cannot be made. For example, the use of "forcing functions" is helpful, as when computerized systems are designed in such a way as to prevent entry of an order for a lethal overdose of a drug.
- *Standardize tasks.* An effective means of reducing error is standardizing processes wherever possible. If a task is done the same way every time—by everyone—there is less chance for error.
- *Reduce the number of hand-offs.* Many errors come from slips in transfers of materials, information, people, instructions, and/or supplies. Processes with fewer hand-offs reduce the chances for such slips.

The system and task redesigns suggested above could serve as the basis for improving the inadequate processes that led to the unnecessary surgery event described at the beginning of this chapter. The following specific corrective actions would likely be effective in decreasing the possibility of future adverse patient occurrences caused by latent failures in the system that cared for Murphy and Jenkins:

- *Reduce reliance on memory.* In reverting to alternative procedures when patients were not wearing identification bands, the staff had to remember to ask patients their identity. Strictly applied protocols for patient care treatment and diagnostic testing would incorporate the step of checking patients' ID bands and would not allow informal variations from this requirement.
- *Improve information access.* The case illustrated many gaps in information communication (for example, patient identity, clinical

information, and practitioner performance data). Systems for generating a patient ID band need improvement. Health information management systems designed to permit access to clinical information by all appropriate practitioners may have helped the radiologist identify the error. Appropriate methods for collecting and trending practitioner performance data are also needed in addition to changing the punitive culture associated with the peer review process.

- *Error-proof processes.* Systems could be created to force the critical task of producing the patient ID band *before* care can proceed. For example, the computerized order entry system could be designed in such a way that it would not accept an order without insertion of a unique code produced when the band is made. A point-of-care bar coding system on the ID band could also be a constraining force.

- *Standardize tasks.* The process in the approved hospital procedures required the checking of patient ID bands, but when the system for producing bands failed, the staff reverted to unapproved alternatives that were more prone to error (for example, questioning the patient to confirm identity, questioning whomever else was around).

- *Reduce the number of hand-offs.* By constructing a flow diagram of the steps of the ED admission process and related patient care activities, unnecessarily complex steps might be discovered. It is important to eliminate as many hand-offs as possible in order to prevent errors in the transfer of patients and information among caregivers.

Health care professionals also need to be taught that safe practice is as important as effective practice. The staff involved in this unnecessary surgery event should have been made aware of the process steps that are essential to safe practice, which would have made them less likely to circumvent these safety-critical steps.

CONCLUSION

Health care professionals are entrusted with people's lives, and when they make a mistake, someone may suffer indeterminate harm or death.

This is a great burden that no true professional takes lightly. Professionals are socialized to be infallible, and when they fail or make a mistake, they face emotional devastation.

How does the same system that has placed professionals on this pedestal respond to an individual's mistakes? It accuses, ostracizes, sanctions, and sues the person involved. After all, how can an error have occurred without negligence? Regulators and accrediting agencies ask health care organizations to report adverse events, and when they do self-report, they are punished with probation or even worse consequences. Is it any wonder then that practitioners conceal their mistakes or try to shift blame?

Patient safety improvements will only come about when leaders in health care organizations and the professionals providing care accept the notion that error is "an inevitable accompaniment of the human condition, even among conscientious professionals with high standards."[37] The very institutions that educate and regulate these clinicians must be the primary change agents for this new attitude. Once we all agree that complete elimination of errors is beyond our control, then we can direct our improvement energies at changing the systems in which humans work.

Changes in attitudes and practices won't come overnight. People do not easily revise well-worn habits of thoughts and deeds. The physicist Max Planck wrote: "A new scientific truth does not triumph by convincing its opponents and making them see the light, but rather because its opponents eventually die, and a new generation grows up that is familiar with it."[38] The medical profession was issued an unprecedented challenge in May 1996 by the American Medical Association when this group announced that "it's time to acknowledge that medical mistakes happen—are even common."[39] There is compelling evidence from the work under way in other complex industries that many medical errors can be eliminated with systems redesign and improved teamwork and through the sheer willpower of people willing to make it happen.[40] Unfortunately, there are no single fixes or magic bullets. Rather, the research reveals a set of factors involved in failure and shows that there are multiple directions for improvements that need to be coordinated in order to make progress on patient safety.[41] To uphold our professional commitment to "first do no harm," we must now begin pursuing each and every one of these new directions.

References and Note

1. Although this case scenario is based on true events from many years ago, it does not involve an actual incident in any hospital currently among those with which the authors associate. Also, the details of the event have been materially altered to protect confidentiality, including use of fictitious names.

2. R. Voelker. "'Treat Systems, Not Errors', Experts Say," *JAMA* 276, no. 19 (November 20, 1996): 1537.

3. L. B. Andrews et al. "An Alternative Strategy for Studying Adverse Events in Medical Care," *Lancet* 349, no. 9048 (February 1, 1997): 309–13.

4. J. Reason. "The Contribution of Latent Human Failures in the Breakdown of Complex Systems," *Philos Trans R Soc Lond* 327B (1990): 476.

5. National Patient Safety Foundation. *A Tale of Two Stories: Contrasting Views of Patient Safety* (Chicago: NPSF, 1998), p. 1, report from a workshop on Assembling the Scientific Basis for Progress on Patient Safety (December 1997). WWW document: URL: http://www.npsf.org/exec.front.html.

6. Cox News Service. "Medical Accident Cited in Boy's Death," *St. Petersburg Times* (January 12, 1996): 1B.

7. M. Wilson. "Surgical horrors," *Chicago Tribune* (March 10, 1995): news p. 7

8. R. A. Knox and D. Golden. "Drug Dosage Was Questioned: Dana-Farber Pharmacist Sent Order Back to Doctor in Breast Cancer Case," *The Boston Globe* (June 19, 1995): metro/region p. 1.

9. A. Fegelman. "U. of C. Cancer Patient Dies of Chemotherapy Overdose," *Chicago Tribune* (June 15, 1995): Chicagoland p. 2.

10. R. Sullivan. "Hospital Admits Fault in Patient's Death," *New York Times* (March 24, 1987): sect B p. 3.

11. M. Romano. "Baby Dies after Injection: Police, State Probe Death at St. Anthony Hospital North," *Rocky Mountain News* (October 24, 1996): local, ed F, p. 5A.

12. S. Twedt. "Despite All His Precautions, an Error Killed His Mother," *Pittsburgh Post-Gazette* (October 28, 1993): national, p. A13.

13. L. Leape. "Error in Medicine," *JAMA* 272, no. 23 (December 21, 1994): 4.

14. J. Reason. *Managing the Risks of Organizational Accidents* (Brookfield, VT: Ashgate Publishing Co., 1997), p. 127.

15. Ibid., p. 128.

16. L. Leape et al. "Systems Analysis of Adverse Drug Events," *JAMA* 274, no. 1 (July 5, 1995): 35.

17. S. E. Feldman and D. W. Roblin. "Medical Accidents in Hospital Care: Applications of Failure Analysis to Hospital Quality Appraisal," *Joint Commission Journal on Quality Improvement* 23, no. 11 (November 1997): p. 569.

18. L. Leape. "Error in Medicine," p. 8.

19. J. Reason. *Managing the Risks of Organizational Accidents*, p. 129.

20. Ibid.

21. National Patient Safety Foundation. *A Tale of Two Stories*, p. 1.

22. D. L. Welch. "Human Error and Human Factors Engineering in Health Care," *Biomedical Instrumentation and Technology* 31, no. 6 (November/December 1997): 627–31.

23. J. B. Cooper, R. S. Newbower, C. D. Long, and B. McPeek. "Preventable Anaesthesia Mishaps: A Study of Human Factors," *Anesthesiology* 49, no. 6 (December 1978): 399–406.

24. M. Currie, D. A. Pybus, and T. A. Torda. "A Prospective Survey of Anaesthetic Critical Events: A Report on a Pilot Study of 88 Cases," *Anaesth Intens Care* 16, no. 1 (February 1988): 103–7.

25. J. B. Cooper, R. S. Newbower, and R. J. Kitz. "An Analysis of Major Errors and Equipment Failures in Anesthesia Management: Considerations for Prevention and Detection," *Anesthesiology* 60, no. 1 (January 1984): 34–42.

26. R. A. Caplan et al. "Adverse Respiratory Events in Anaesthesia: A Closed Claims Analysis," *Anesthesiology* 72 no. 5 (May 1990): 828–33.

27. M. E. PatJ-Cornell. "Risk Analysis Model Targets Anesthesia Incidents," *Anesthesia Patient Safety Foundation Newsletter* 7, no. 2 (Summer 1992): 1–10.

28. D. M. Gaba, K. J. Fish, and S. K. Howard. *Crisis Management in Anesthesiology* (New York: Churchill Livingstone, 1994), pp. 1–294.

29. J. H. Van der Walt et al. "Recovery Room Incidents in the First 2000 Incident Reports," *Anaesth Intens Care* 21, no. 5 (October 1993): 650–52.

30. J. A. Williamson et al. "Human Failure: An Analysis of 2000 Incident Reports," *Anaesth Intens Care* 21, no. 5 (October 1993): 678–83.

31. W. J. Russell et al. "Problems with Ventilation: An Analysis of 2000 Incident Reports," *Anaesth Intens Care* 21, no. 5 (October 1993): 617–20.

32. G. L. Zeitlin. "Possible Decrease in Mortality Associated with Anesthesia. A Comparison of Two Time Periods in Massachusetts, USA," *Anaesthesia* 44, no. 5 (May 1989): 432–33.

33. L. Leape, "Error in Medicine," pp. 12–13.

34. L. L. Leape et al. *Reducing Adverse Drug Events* (Boston: Institute for Healthcare Improvement, 1998).

35. R. I. Cook and D. D. Woods. "Operating at the Sharp End: The Complexity of Human Error," in M. S. Bogner, ed., *Human Error in Medicine* (Hinsdale, NJ: Lawrence Erlbaum, 1994): 255–310.

36. Institute for Healthcare Improvement. "The Quest for Error-Proof Medicine," *Drug Benefit Trends* 9, no. 6 (1997): 18, 23, 27–29.

37. L. Leape. "Error in Medicine," p. 14.

38. M. L. Millenson. *Citing Max Planck, Demanding Medical Excellence: Doctors and Accountability in the Information Age* (Chicago: University of Chicago Press, 1997): 367.

39. L. O. Prager. "Safety-Centered Care," *American Medical News* 36, no. 26 (May 13, 1996): 1.

40. M. L. Millenson. *Citing Max Planck*, p. 73.

41. National Patient Safety Foundation. *A Tale of Two Stories*, p. 13.

2

Measuring Performance of High-Risk Processes

Karen Ferraco
Patrice L. Spath, BA, ART

M anagement of errors in complex organizations, according to James Reason, has two components: error containment and error reduction.[1] Error containment consists of the actions taken to limit adverse consequences once an incident happens, while error reduction consists of actions taken to limit the occurrence of errors. Unlike many of the chapters in this book that deal primarily with error containment strategies, this chapter describes an important component of error reduction: performance measurement of high-risk processes. Such evaluations can provide an organization with vital information about the incidence of errors as well as insights into the error-producing factors that may ultimately lead to a harmful incident.

Health care performance measures can be used to evaluate many aspects of quality (for example, appropriateness of resource use, financial viability, clinical outcomes, effectiveness of treatment, and so on). This chapter focuses primarily on measures related to medical errors, although many of the traditional quality measures can serve a dual purpose. For example, hospital cancer programs annually report the number of new cancer cases and stage at time of diagnosis. A common quality of care measure is "Percent of new breast cancer cases diagnosed as Stage 0 (in situ) or Stage 1 (localized) at time of diagnosis."[2] This performance measure helps the organization identify access and patient management problems. However, failure to identify suspicious breast lesions is a significant risk management concern for primary care physicians as well as radiologists. Failure to correctly and rapidly arrive at the right diagnosis can lead to an adverse patient outcome and may increase the chance of patient injury and subsequent legal action.

The purpose of performance measurement in error management is to discover, assess, and correct problem areas before a significant untoward patient incident occurs. Traditionally, individual case studies of events resulting in patient injury have been the primary source of information about medical errors. These case reviews can be extremely useful as educational and analytic tools. By evaluating the circumstances surrounding an event, clinicians may identify sources and causes of poor outcomes, which may in turn result in immediate behavioral or process changes. However, organizations cannot rely solely on case-by-case analysis to ensure the safety of high-risk processes. Common patient safety problems will not be identified and corrected if the focus of review is only on disastrous events that largely occur randomly and can only be examined after the fact. Retrospective case-by-case review must be supplemented by ongoing monitoring of safety-critical steps in high-risk processes. Regular analysis of the performance of high-risk processes provides the organization with a snapshot view of the number of failed safety-critical steps that have a high potential for grievous consequences. The data are used to identify and change undesirable practices that increase the chance of patient injury.

Error management in health care is a multidimensional endeavor. This chapter delves into the different approaches of performance measurement and provides the reader with examples of the various types and sources of data that can be used in a patient safety improvement initiative. To achieve error reduction goals, the measurement data must be reported and analyzed. Described in this chapter are various techniques for evaluating error management data using internal analysis and external benchmarking strategies.

MONITOR HIGH-RISK PROCESSES

The quantity and quality of all patient care processes should be subjected to some type of evaluation. However, there are so many disciplines, technical procedures, and individual decisions made in health care that it is economically impossible to measure all aspects. Therefore, measures must be focused on high-risk processes. In the context of this chapter, a high-risk process is defined as any health care delivery activity that (1) has a high probability of error; (2) occurs with sufficient frequency; or (3) would result in severe patient injury if an error is made. From a risk management perspective, high-risk processes would be considered those activities that have the highest exposure for financial loss to the organization.[3]

The determination of what is a high-risk process is somewhat dependent on the health care setting and services provided. Analysis of malpractice claims data has shown certain activities to be associated with a greater risk of patient injury. These include the following:[4-7]

- Diagnostic and therapeutic decision making
- Patient assessment/observation (by physicians, nurses, and other caregivers)
- Transfer of patient care responsibilities between caregivers and facilities
- Communication (among caregivers and between caregivers and patients)
- Monitoring of patients during and immediately following high-risk interventions (for example, procedures performed under anesthesia or restraint/seclusion)
- Medication administration (prescribing, preparing, and dispensing medications) and monitoring their effects

Most people would agree that malpractice claims are merely the tip of the iceberg. However, the data derived from claims analysis serve as one more piece of evidence that organizations can use in selecting the risk-prone activities that should be constantly monitored for performance problems.

High-Risk Patient Groups

The patient population being cared for in the organization or by the individual clinician can have an impact on the riskiness of health care activities. For example:

- Andrews and her colleagues found that the seriousness of a patient's underlying illness was linked to an increased likelihood of an initial adverse event in a hospital.[8] The researchers also found that patients with long hospital stays had more adverse events, with the likelihood of a patient experiencing an adverse event increasing about 6 percent for each day of hospitalization. A similar relationship between long hospital stays, patient comorbidities, and iatrogenic events was noted by Lefevre and colleagues.[9]

- The acuity of hospitalized patients has been shown to positively correlate with undesirable occurrences such as pressure ulcers, infections, and deaths.[10]
- In-hospital patient injury is generally associated with host factors long known to promote falls: increasing age, debility/decreased functioning, and central nervous system depressant medication.[11]
- The patient under treatment for depression or other psychiatric conditions may also be at higher risk of an untoward incident as evidenced by the sentinel event database of the Joint Commission on Accreditation of Healthcare Organizations (Joint Commission). By December 1998 the Joint Commission's Accreditation Committee had reviewed 80 cases of inpatient suicides.[12]
- Patients with autoimmune deficiencies or those who cannot easily recover from the physical assault of a clinical error or mishap (for example, neonatal patients, patients receiving chemotherapy, severely ill or frail elderly patients) are also at high risk for adverse events.[13,14]

High-Risk Activities

Some health care processes are well established as high-risk activities regardless of the patient populations being served. For example, many aspects of medication use have a high risk potential for lethal errors. In the Harvard Medical Practice Study, researchers reported that drug-related incidents were the most common adverse events in hospitalized patients.[15] In a nine-year study at one teaching hospital, antimicrobials, cardiovascular agents, gastrointestinal agents, and narcotics were found to be the most common medication classes involved in errors.[16] When the tasks of generating and filling prescriptions as well as administration of medication are not performed as required, significant patient harm has been known to occur.

Even in the outpatient setting, medication use has been shown to be a predictor of patient safety problems. For example, an informal survey of nonhospitalized veterans conducted by the Australian Department of Veterans Affairs found that those who had more than 20 dispensings of medications over the previous six months were at high risk for medication-related problems (for example, misunderstanding of dosage instructions, adverse reactions, medication duplication, overdose, and so on).[17] A similar study conducted in the United States at the Durham Veterans Affairs Medical Center found that 58 percent of 167 older outpatients who were taking five or more scheduled medications experienced a confirmed adverse drug event.[18]

Measuring performance of medication use should include global measures (incidence of medication errors) as well as focused measures that evaluate aspects of "high-alert" medication use. Examples of high-alert medications that are known to be associated with adverse events are listed below:[19]

- *Medications with similar names.* For example, in one incident a physician ordered ketoralac for a 10-year-old child after surgery but the pharmacy dispensed three vials of Ketalar instead. Luckily, the child's nurse noticed the error and the correct drug was then dispensed.
- *Medications with similar packaging.* For example, in a recent incident, a nurse prepared an epidural infusion for a postpartum cesarean section mother using two vials of gentamicin instead of the fentanyl that was ordered. Both the gentamicin and fentanyl vials had look-alike red flip tops. Fortunately the patient did not develop toxicity symptoms after inadvertently receiving 160 mg of gentamicin.
- *Medications that are not commonly used or prescribed.* For example, in one tragic case a nurse was charged with the responsibility of providing Actinomycin-D to a patient with Wilm's tumor. Because she had never before administered this drug and was unfamiliar with its normal dosage levels, she inadvertently transposed the dosage from 2.7 mg to 7.2 mg, which resulted in the death of a 32-year-old patient.
- *Commonly used medications (for example, antibiotics, opiates, and NSAIDS) to which many patients are allergic.* In one incident, penicillin was ordered for a patient who was allergic to

that medication. However, the clinic office staff had mistakenly documented the allergy on the record of the patient's son. The patient did not recognize the drug's name as a penicillin derivative and he nearly died when he took it.

- *Medications (lithium, warfarin, digoxin, theophylline) that require testing to ensure that proper therapeutic levels are achieved.* A recent case involved an elderly man who was on coumadin following hip replacement. Because the man's coumadin levels were not adequately monitored, he developed an acute pulmonary embolus.

The standards of the Joint Commission suggest that medication use as well as other important health care activities be regularly evaluated in an organization's performance improvement program. Listed in figure 2-1 are the areas in which organizations are expected to concentrate performance measurement activities in 1999.[20] Some of these measurement data may be used to identify or monitor high-risk processes.

Once an organization identifies the high-risk processes that should be regularly evaluated, the next step is to define the measures that will be used in this evaluation. Some of the measures may already be in place within the organization's risk management or performance improvement program. In other instances it will be necessary to identify additional measures to strengthen the error-reduction initiative.

MEASURE PERFORMANCE

Good health care performance requires providing services that are appropriate for each patient's condition; providing them safely, competently,

Figure 2-1.   Activities That Must Be Regularly Evaluated in Health Care Organizations Accredited by the Joint Commission

- Operative and other procedures that place patients at risk
- Use of blood and blood components
- Medication use
- Patient restraint and seclusion
- Care provided to high-risk populations
- Management of the environment of care
- Needs, expectations, and satisfaction of patients

and in an appropriate time frame; and achieving desired outcomes.[21] A performance measure is some form of a rate, ratio, or proportion that can be used as a tool to evaluate one or more of these aspects of health care services. A common method of creating such a measurement is to identify a group of patients who received care during a given "time window" and then determine how many of those patients received "good" service. Patients who received good quality of care are counted in the numerator of the performance rate or score. A measure of bad performance can be constructed similarly by counting patients who did not receive good quality of care in the numerator.

Performance measures can also be used to evaluate the quality of specific health care processes. For example, the number of medications prescribed during a given time window can be compared with the number of prescription errors during that same time period. The population under study by this performance measure is prescriptions, not patients.

Performance measurement is an activity that has long been required by government regulators of the health care industry as well as by voluntary accreditation organizations. Performance measures are now being used to assess a wide variety of health care activities. If these same yardsticks are also to be used to identify sources of exposure in high-risk processes, choosing the right performance measure is an important step. The ultimate purpose of patient safety performance measures is to reduce the number of avoidable patient injuries and deaths. To achieve this purpose, safety-related performance measures must be like the canary in the coal mine, providing a reliable early warning of safety-related problems.

Errors that result in actual significant injury to patients, clients, or residents are easily identified after the fact. The difficulty lies in the identification of patterns of near-miss behavior—those actions that did not result in a patient's death or serious physical or psychological injury but which, under different conditions or with additional failures, could have caused such an outcome. At this time there is no industrywide consensus about what are near-miss behaviors to measure or how to measure them. Therefore, health care entities are left to themselves to determine which performance measures will be used to identify error-producing factors that need further investigation.

Two types of performance measures can be used to identify failures in high-risk processes. These are process measures and outcome measures. Process measures provide information about whether or not people are "doing the right things." Outcome measures provide information about whether or not people are "doing the right things well."[22]

Process Measures

The provision of health care, whether in an inpatient or outpatient environment, involves a multitude of activities. The performance of any number of these activities can be measured. When selecting patient safety-related measures, be sure to concentrate evaluation efforts on those elements that are likely to affect the safe delivery of health care services.

Process measures can be used to evaluate what Donebedian called the structure or characteristics of the care setting.[23] Measures of the safety-related structural components would be used to evaluate performance in areas such as the following:

- Compliance with safety regulations and codes
- Adequacy of equipment maintenance
- Physician and staff certification, training, and continuing education
- Oversight of physician and staff competency
- Workplace ergonomics
- Staff scheduling
- Telecommunications and information systems

Other safety-related process measures would be used to monitor the incidence of variations from accepted policies, regulations, and standards of practice that could potentially result in patient harm. The number of medication errors that occur in a facility is a common process measure. A medication error is any variation from an expected process that may cause or lead to inappropriate medication use or patient harm. For example, a physician ordering an incorrect dose of a medication would be considered a variation from the "right" process (appropriate drug ordering). While the error may be caught and corrected before patient harm occurs, a process variance has still occurred.

Researchers recently coined the term *adverse event* to describe a situation in which an inappropriate decision (action or inaction) was made when, at the time, an appropriate alternative could have been chosen.[24] Data about the number of adverse events (using this definition) would tell caregivers how well the clinical decision-making process is work-ing. These data would not measure the outcome of that process.

Outcome Measures

Outcomes represent the cumulative effect of health care processes on patients. An example of an outcome measure of patient safety is the num-ber of patient falls. Although caregivers may have followed the right process, something caused the patient to experience a fall. Counts of serious events would also be considered outcome measures. For exam-ple, an event involving a medical product is defined as serious by the Food and Drug Administration (FDA) MedWatch Program if any of the following outcomes occurred as a result of using a medical product:[25]

- Patient's death is suspected as being a direct outcome of the adverse event.
- Patient was at substantial risk of dying or it was suspected that the use or continued use of the product would result in the patient's death.
- Patient required admission to the hospital or hospitalization was prolonged because of the adverse event.
- Patient experienced a significant, persistent, or permanent change, impairment, damage, or disruption in his or her body function/structure, physical activities, or quality of life.
- Patient was exposed to a medical product prior to conception or during pregnancy that resulted in an adverse outcome in the child.
- Patient developed a condition that required medical or surgical intervention to preclude permanent impairment or damage.

The Joint Commission uses the phrase *sentinel event* to describe a serious event. A sentinel event is considered an unexpected occurrence involving death or serious physical or psychological injury or the risk thereof. The phrase *risk thereof* includes any process variation for which a recurrence would carry a significant chance of a serious adverse outcome.[26] A measure of the number of sentinel events is an outcome measure. These data do not necessarily tell caregivers how well they are doing at following the right processes; however, it does provide information about how many serious events actually occur.

A comprehensive error reduction initiative should include both process and outcome measures. Listed in figure 2-2 are examples of common process and outcome measures that would be useful for identifying error-related problems in various types of facilities. The data from these measures could be reported for the organization as a whole and could also be stratified by individual departments or services.

The measures in figure 2-2 are broad measures that offer a "snapshot" of the organization's patient safety performance. Although global measures of process and outcome such as these provide an overview of the incidence of errors or bad outcomes, these measures may not be sufficiently sensitive to provide early warnings of impending disasters. It is recommended that global measures be supplemented with measures that evaluate compliance with safety-critical tasks.

Measuring Safety-Critical Tasks

It is cost prohibitive to measure every aspect of a high-risk process. Therefore, it is important to identify those tasks in the process that are critical to patient safety and should be regularly examined. A safety-critical task is one that must be done properly all of the time.[27] If a safety-critical task is performed incorrectly, the error could lead to catastrophic results. While not all such errors will cause patient injury or death, serious mistakes in high-risk processes can start an accident chain of events that may be difficult to stop in certain circumstances. The criticality of a task in a high-risk process can be expressed as:

Level of risk × likelihood of occurrence = task criticality

The level of risk refers to the amount of damage expected when a failure occurs at this step in the process. In this instance, damage refers to the severity of patient injury. For example, an incorrect overdose prescription of a chemotherapy agent that is not caught before the drug is administered is more likely to cause patient harm than the same error occurring in the prescription of a less toxic drug. The likelihood of occurrence refers to the estimated frequency of such errors happening. This prediction can be based on past performance measurement results or it may represent an educated guess by those intimately involved in the process.

Figure 2-2.   General Risk-Related Performance Measures

Acute Care Services

- Percent of records with adequately documented informed consent (organization to define "adequate")
- Percent of consultations completed as requested or within 24 hours
- Percent of new admissions seen by primary physician within 12 hours
- Number of unplanned transfers to special care unit (intensive care, coronary care, neonatal intensive care, etc.)
- Percent of patients who are unexpectedly admitted or retained following a complication of outpatient surgery or anesthesia event
- Number of unplanned readmissions within 48 hours
- Number of delayed diagnoses (organization to define "delayed")
- Number of missed diagnoses (organization to define "missed")
- Number of cases in which a significant change in the patient's condition or diagnosis did not result in a reassessment (organization to define "significant")
- Number of unplanned patient returns to the operating room
- Number of adverse events occurring during anesthesia use (including conscious sedation)
- Percent of patients who expire within 30 days following surgical procedure (excludes deaths due to normal course of patient's disease)
- Percent of records in which all treatments/visits are recorded
- Percent of cases in which attending physician was promptly notified about out-of-range or unusual diagnostic test results (organization to define "prompt notification")
- Number or percent of patients developing complications (organization to define reportable complications)
- Rate of nosocomial infections
- Percent of cases in which there is a documented response to consultants' suggestions
- Percent of live births entering intermediate or intensive care nurseries
- In-hospital mortality rate for low birth-weight babies
- Perinatal mortality rate
- Number of patient suicides (attempted/successful)
- Patients admitted following attempted suicide for whom there is no documented suicide prevention plan
- Percent of patients at suicide risk who receive appropriate consultation prior to a leave of absence (organization to define "appropriate")
- Percent of patients who are adequately searched after returning from leave of absence (organization to define "adequate")
- Percent of locked units with adequate security (organization to define "adequate")

(Continued on next page)

Figure 2-2.   (Continued)

- Percent of patients in restraint/seclusion who are adequately monitored (organization to define "adequate")
- Ratio of patient restraint/seclusion hours to patient days
- Ratio of medication errors to medications dispensed or administered
- Ratio of potential adverse drug events to number of medications ordered (a potential adverse drug event is a serious medication error that had the potential to harm the patient but, either by luck or interception, did not)
- Percent of patients who develop an adverse drug reaction
- Percent of patients undergoing procedure requiring isotope injection who develop an adverse reaction to the isotope agent
- Ratio of transfusion reactions to total units transfused
- Ratio of patient falls to patient days
- Number of serious patient injuries/deaths that may have been related to the use of a medical device
- Percent of fire alarms/protection equipment tested as required
- Percent of new devices/equipment added to inventory only after relevant physicians/staff have received in-service training
- Percent of equipment maintenance checks completed within required time frame (organization to define requirements)
- Percent of emergency generator tests that cause a major interruption in patient care activities (organization to define "major interruption")
- Percent of staff who demonstrate adequate knowledge of their roles in internal/external disaster situations
- Percent of hazard surveillance surveys completed within required time frame
- Percent of significant hazards identified through surveillance that are resolved within acceptable time frame (organization to define "significant hazard" and "acceptable time frame")
- Number of open and pending liability claims

Long-Term Care Services

- Number of cases in which a significant change in the patient's condition or diagnosis did not result in a reassessment (organization to define "significant")
- Percent of residents who experience an unplanned weight loss problem (5 percent change in 30 days or 10 percent change in 180 days)
- Percent of cases in which attending physician was promptly notified about out-of-range or unusual diagnostic test results (organization to define "prompt notification")
- Number or percent of residents developing complications (organization to define reportable complications)
- Rate of nosocomial infections
- Percent of residents who develop a pressure ulcer at Stage II or higher, when no ulcers were previously present at Stage II or higher

Figure 2-2.   (Continued)

- Number of resident suicides (attempted/successful)
- Number of resident elopements
- Ratio of resident restraint/seclusion hours to resident days
- Ratio of medication errors to medications dispensed or administered
- Ratio of potential adverse drug events to number of medications ordered (a potential adverse drug event is a serious medication error that had the potential to harm the resident but, either by luck or interception, did not)
- Percent of residents who develop an adverse drug reaction
- Ratio of resident falls to resident days
- Number of serious resident injuries/deaths that may have been related to the use of a medical device
- Percent of fire alarms/protection equipment tested as required
- Percent of new devices/equipment added to inventory only after relevant physicians/staff have received in-service training
- Percent of equipment maintenance checks completed within required time frame (organization to define requirements)
- Percent of emergency generator tests that cause a major interruption in patient care activities (organization to define "major interruption")
- Percent of staff who demonstrate adequate knowledge of their roles in internal/external disaster situations
- Percent of hazard surveillance surveys completed within required time frame
- Percent of significant hazards identified through surveillance that are resolved within acceptable time frame (organization to define "significant hazard" and "acceptable time frame")
- Number of open and pending liability claims

Home Health Services

- Percent of clients on home IV therapy who require hospital admission
- Percent of clients on ventilators who develop respiratory infection
- Percent of cases with documentation of adequate patient education regarding home safety (organization to define "adequate")
- Percent of cases with documented evidence that the physician remains involved in the care of the patient (organization to define "documented evidence")
- Percent of clients failing to meet functional health status goals without evidence of care plan assessment and revision
- Ratio of medication errors to medications administered
- Number of adverse drug reactions
- Number of serious client injuries/deaths that may have been related to the use of a medical device

(Continued on next page)

Figure 2-2.   (Continued)

- Percent of clients developing complications following venipuncture (hemolyzed specimens, hematoma, infection, etc.)
- Number of mislabeled/misplaced specimens obtained by caregiver during home visit
- Number of times that client records are missing/unavailable at time of scheduled home visit
- Percent of abnormal diagnostic results or physical findings not communicated to physician within established time frames
- Percent of clients developing new contractures or pressure sores while receiving rehabilitation therapy
- Percent of clients referred to the appropriate treatment program (organization to define treatment appropriateness criteria for different conditions)

Ambulatory Services

- Number of patients who return to clinic within 72 hours due to failure to improve
- Number of missed appointments for high-risk patients (organization to define "high risk")
- Number of patients who are noncompliant with medications without evidence of caregiver intervention
- Percent of patients on more than five prescribed medications without evidence of medication counseling
- Number of medication-prescribing errors
- Percent of patient records lacking notation of allergies (or "no known allergies")
- Number of outdated medications in medication supply area
- Number of misplaced/misfiled/misidentified laboratory or radiographic findings
- Number of instances in which laboratory results fell outside established quality control limits and no verification of findings was done
- Percent of patients developing complications following venipuncture (hemolyzed specimens, hematoma, infection, etc.)
- Percent of patients who are unexpectedly retained following a complication of outpatient procedure or anesthesia event
- Number of mislabeled/misplaced specimens
- Number of serious patient injuries/deaths that may have been related to the use of a medical device
- Percent of scheduled appointments at which patient's record was missing/ unavailable at the time of the clinic visit
- Number of patient encounters (visit or telephone) not documented in record
- Number of open and pending liability claims

The matrix in table 2-1 illustrates how this criticality scoring system can be used to choose the tasks that should be regularly monitored for a high-risk process such as administration of warfarin. The tasks of the process are listed in stepwise fashion in the first column. A numeric risk score and frequency score are assigned to each task. The criticality score for each task is calculated by multiplying the risk score times the frequency score. The highest possible task criticality score is 16. Organizations should consider regularly monitoring the performance of any task that has a criticality score of 8 or higher to ensure that problems in this safety-critical step are quickly identified and resolved. Examples of performance measures that can be used to evaluate various safety-critical steps are listed in figure 2-3. These measures are sorted into the major patient care functions identified by the Joint Commission's accreditation standards and relevant sites of care.

It is not necessary or desirable for organizations to use all of the global measures listed in figure 2-2 or gather measurement data for every safety-critical task. Collecting as much information as possible about patient safety can result in paralysis. It is much better to work with only a few measures that you understand and know how to use. It is also important to periodically evaluate your choice of risk-related measures to determine if changes or additions are needed.

COLLECT MEASUREMENT DATA

A challenge in any performance measurement effort is the data collection process. To ensure that valid information is gathered it is important to identify reliable data sources. Various handwritten documents and computerized databases can be used to collect data for the numerator, denominator, and other data elements necessary to calculate the measure. Many factors affect the choice of a data source for a particular performance measure. The considerations include the following:

- What information is contained in the data source
- The accuracy and reliability of the data
- Which patients and processes are covered by the data
- The costs involved in capturing the data
- Whether the data are computerized or manually recorded
- The timeliness of the data

Table 2-1. Task Criticality Scoring System for the Process of Warfarin Administration

Process Tasks	Risk Level[a]	Likelihood of Failure[b]	Task Criticality Score (risk level × likelihood of failure)
Physician writes warfarin medication order.			
Nurse reviews order and clarifies it if necessary.			
Order is transcribed to medication administration record (MAR).			
Order is transmitted to pharmacy.			
Pharmacist reviews order and clarifies it if necessary.			
Drug is prepared and dispensed.			
Drug is delivered to nursing unit.			
Nurse matches drug to MAR; variations are clarified with pharmacy and/or physician.			
Nurse prepares to administer drug (checks "Five Rights").			
Nurse administers drug to patient.			
Medication administration is charted.			
Patient's response is monitored.			

[a]Risk-Level Scoring Key:

   4 = Catastrophic (failure of this task could cause loss of patient life or permanent impairment)
   3 = Serious (failure could cause severe patient injury or temporary disability)
   2 = Minor (failure could cause minor patient injury)
   1 = Negligible (failure is unlikely to cause patient injury)

[b]Likelihood of Occurrence Scoring Key:

   4 = Probable (failure of this task occurs frequently)
   3 = Occasional (failure occurs sporadically)
   2 = Rare (failure is very uncommon, but it does happen)
   1 = Improbable (failure has never been known to occur)

Figure 2-3.   Examples of Performance Measures for Safety-Critical Tasks in Major Patient Care Functions

Operative and other procedures

Acute and ambulatory surgery

- Percent of cases in which correct patient/surgical site was confirmed prior to start of operation (as required by policies/procedures)
- Percent of cases requiring sponge/needle counts in which full count sheet is completed correctly
- Percent of cases requiring sponge/needle counts with reported discrepancy
- Percent of patients experiencing hypotension when receiving IV sedation
- Percent of patients experiencing loss of sensation due to position during anesthesia
- Percent of patients experiencing cardiac-related problems during withdrawal from general anesthesia
- Percent of cases cancelled after patient has entered operating room holding area
- Percent of surgeries performed without history and physical examination present in patient's record
- Percent of patients who experience a cardiac arrest within two postprocedure days of procedures involving anesthesia administration
- Percent of surgeries delayed or cancelled due to unavailable or incomplete equipment/supplies
- Percent of procedures in which there is a break in sterile techniques
- Percent of total pathological specimens removed in the operating room that are lost or mislabeled

Behavioral health care

- Percent of patients undergoing electroshock therapy (ECT) without pre-ECT workup, which includes: dental consultation, skull and spinal column x-ray studies, and electrocardiogram

Medication usage

Acute, emergent, and ambulatory care

- Percent of patients who experience extravasation during administration of chemotherapy
- Percent of inpatients on heparin and coumadin therapy whose prothrombin times are not monitored according to approved guidelines
- Percent of patients on warfarin whose prothrombin times are maintained at 1.5–2.0 times the control value
- Percent of outpatients on anticoagulants who do not have at least one prothrombin time test done every 30 days
- Percent of high-risk surgery patients for whom deep vein thrombosis prophylactic measures/treatment are not implemented
- Percent of patients receiving pitocin without adequate documentation of the indications for use
- Percent of medication orders requiring clarification because of illegibility

(Continued on next page)

Figure 2-3.   (Continued)

- Percent of medication orders containing "nonapproved" abbreviations or acronyms
- Percent of medication orders containing dosing that is incorrect for patient age or condition
- Percent of patients on potassium whose plasma levels are greater than about 5 (exact level to be determined by organization)
- Percent of diabetic patients whose glucose plasma levels are less than about 50 (exact level to be determined by organization)
- Percent of patients receiving IV sedation in the emergency department (ED) who are released to appropriate family/significant other and instructed not to drive
- Percent of cases in which information about patient's home medications is available to treating physician
- Percent of patients admitted through the ED with a principal diagnosis of acute myocardial infarction who receive thrombolytic therapy
- Average time from admission to the ED to administration of thrombolytic therapy for patients with a principal diagnosis of acute myocardial infarction
- Percent of inpatients receiving digoxin who have no corresponding measured drug level or whose highest measured level exceeds a specified limit
- Percent of inpatients receiving theophylline who have no corresponding measured drug level or whose highest measured level exceeds a specified limit
- Percent of inpatients receiving phenytoin who have no corresponding measured drug level or whose highest measured level exceeds a specified limit
- Percent of outpatients receiving antihypertensives whose potassium levels are below normal
- Percent of patients receiving antibiotics for surgical prophylaxis in which first dose was administered within one hour of surgical incision
- Number of medications administered but not documented

Behavioral health care

- Percent of schizophrenic patients receiving doses of haloperidol or fluphenazine in excess of 20 mg per day
- Percent of patients receiving MAO inhibitors without evidence of dietary monitoring
- Percent of patients on Tegretol who have a complete blood count performed every two months
- Percent of inpatients receiving lithium who have no corresponding measured drug level or whose highest measured level exceeds a specified limit

Skilled/residential care

- Percent of patients regularly receiving more than five medications

Home care

- Percent of clients receiving infusion therapy for whom therapy is discontinued before prescribed completion
- Number of interruptions in infusion therapy

Figure 2-3. (Continued)

Use of blood and blood products

Acute and ambulatory care

- Percent of contaminated units appropriately discarded (according to procedures)
- Number of outdated units in active blood supply
- Percent of patients developing complications from too rapid administration of blood transfusion

Patient rights/organizational ethics

Acute, long-term, home, and ambulatory care

- Percent of patients (or their families/significant others) queried about advance directives on admission
- Percent of patients with advance directives who have a copy of the directive in their medical record
- Percent of patients who refuse evaluation and treatment
- Percent of patients seen in the ED who refuse transport to another facility for treatment
- Percent of patients who change their primary care physician within a specified period
- Percent of patients requiring foreign language or sign-language interpretation who are provided such assistance within specified time frame (as defined by organization's policies)

Patient assessment

Acute care

- Average order-to-report times for critical diagnostic tests (organization to define "critical")
- Percent of cases with abnormal diagnostic test results on admission without corresponding documentation in the patient assessment
- Percent of inpatients with congestive heart failure for whom a weight is obtained on admission and thereafter at least daily
- Percent of orthopedic procedures involving extremities in which descriptive CMS checks are not adequately documented by nursing staff the first 12 hours postop
- Percent of newborn deliveries involving fetal distress in which the response time is 30 minutes or greater from the first sign of distress
- Percent of radiology studies in which pathology identified later was not found on initial study
- Percent of cases in which ED physician's interpretation of x-ray studies differs from radiologist's interpretation
- Percent of patients admitted with a diagnosis of depressive disorder who are not assessed for the potential for harm to both self and others
- Number of patients that develop fluid overload due to inattention to the patient's intravenous line and/or rate of infusion

(Continued on next page)

Figure 2-3. (Continued)

Ambulatory

- Number of patients with a breast mass that does not disappear or become smaller within six weeks of initial discovery (regardless of the mammogram findings) who do not undergo additional diagnostic tests
- Percent of patients with an initial diagnosis of depressive disorder who are not assessed for the potential for harm to both self and others
- Percent of patients with verified hypertension (i.e., blood pressure > 140/90 taken on three occasions during a two-month period) who do not receive hypertensive workup/assessment and follow-up

Home care

- Number of clients who develop aspiration pneumonia who did not have appropriate assessment and referral (organization to define "appropriate")
- Percent of clients who have a home situation that puts them at risk of readmission to the hospital who are not evaluated by a clinical nurse specialist

Care of patients

Acute and emergency care

- Percent of patients identified as having functional needs who have an assessment/intervention by the appropriate therapist (organization to define "functional needs" requiring therapist consultation and "appropriate" therapist)
- Percent of unsuccessful first attempts at orotracheal intubation
- Percent of unsuccessful first attempts at intravenous line insertion
- Percent of patients who develop latex anaphylaxis who have a known history of latex allergy
- Percent of newborn deliveries in which physician/midwife is not in attendance
- Percent of diagnostic tests requiring repeat due to technical error on first examination
- Percent of patients undergoing fracture repair procedure who develop postop dislocation/displacement due to improper positioning
- Percent of vascular grafts/cannulas that become occluded, requiring replacement
- Percent of patients with suspected pulmonary edema who are positioned in high Fowler's position with lower extremities dependent
- Intraoperative mortality of trauma patients with a systolic blood pressure of less than 70mmHg within two hours of ED or inpatient admission who did not undergo a laparotomy or thoracotomy
- Percent of patients with endotracheal tube that develop complications related to cuff overinflation
- Percent of patients that aspirate during a tube feeding

Ambulatory care

- Percent of patients with a diagnosis of intentional drug overdose or other suicidal gesture who are not referred for mental health counseling

Figure 2-3.   (Continued)

- Percent of patients followed through the full term of their pregnancy who have a minimum of five visits or a satisfactory reason for fewer than five visits is documented
- Percent of known diabetic patients who undergo hemoglobin A1c measurement, ophthalmologic exam, and total cholesterol measurement at least annually
- Number of medication or treatment modalities that are not given because the stock is out of date, not available, damaged, or lost
- Percent of indwelling vascular grafts/cannulas that become occluded, requiring replacement

Home care

- Percent of clients with diet-controlled diabetes who receive nutritional counseling
- Percent of clients with two acute episodes of congestive heart failure in a six-month period who are not referred to the cardiopulmonary team

Patient education

Acute, ambulatory, and home care

- Number of readmissions due to insufficient/inadequate patient education on a prior admission
- Percent of cases in which there is documentation that patient/family demonstrated an understanding of postdischarge precautions
- Inpatients with a diagnosis of insulin-dependent diabetes mellitus who demonstrate self-blood glucose monitoring and self-administration of insulin before discharge, or are referred for postdischarge follow-up for diabetes management

Continuum of care

Acute, emergency, ambulatory, and home care

- Percent of patients transferred to another facility from the ED without documentation of stable condition prior to transfer
- Percent of cases in which ED physician's interpretation of x-ray studies differs from radiologist's interpretation and attending physician is not notified of discrepancy
- Percent of home health care cases requiring physician contact (according to agency policy) in which physician was contacted within required time frame
- Percent of patients given IV/IM Demerol, Valium, or other sedatives with no evidence that family or friend drove them home

Behavioral health

- Percent of cases in which a written relapse prevention plan is documented prior to the patient's discharge from inpatient care
- Percent of patients for whom a follow-up appointment is scheduled within two weeks of inpatient discharge

The three basic sources of data are the following:

1. Incident reports (sometimes termed *variance* or *occurrence reports*), the most common source of patient safety-related process and outcome data
2. Administrative data (for example, computerized databases that include enrollment, encounter, or hospital discharge data or malpractice claims files)
3. Patient records (all data stored in a paper or computerized patient record, such as laboratory results, procedure notes, discharge notes, and consultation reports)

The accuracy and completeness of the information in the data source will determine the level of confidence one can have about the measurement results.

Incident Reports

Incident reports have been used as a risk management data source for more than 30 years. Most health care facilities require the staff to fill out an incident report when a variance has occurred from the usual process of patient care. These reports are meant to be nonjudgmental, factual accounts of the event and its consequences, if any. An example of a hospital incident report form is shown in figure 2-4.

Obtaining accurate, valid, and reliable information from incident reports is not without its challenges. Following are the four primary problems found with most incident reporting programs:

1. All incidents may not be reported, depending on people's willingness to report.
2. Data items are not well defined or understood by the staff.
3. Reports lack sufficient detail for effective analysis.
4. Reports may not be completed for all near-miss situations or truly serious events.

The first problem—an individual's willingness to report an incident—is strongly linked to the organizational culture and how the information is used.[28] If the involved staff member is blamed for the event and

Figure 2-4. Sample Hospital Incident Report

INCIDENT REPORT

Complete immediately for every incident
and send to manager

—**Confidential Report of Incident**—
—**Not a Part of the Medical Record**—

(Addressograph or name and address)

Please Print

Patient _____ Age _____ Sex ____ Unit/room _____
　　　　(Last name)　　　　　(First name)

Date of incident _____ Time _____ Physician notified? __ Yes __ No

Physician _____

Physician's response _____

Bed rails up? __ Yes __ No　Safety belt in place? __ Yes __ No

Bed position: __ High __ Low

Exact location of incident _____

Account of incident _____

Signature_____ Date: _____

Department Manager's Action:

List of persons involved or familiar with incident:

Name: _____

Name: _____

Classification of Incident
(Check one that most closely defines)

__ Fall without injury　　__ Medication error
__ Fall with injury　　　 __ Missed dose/order
__ Fracture/dislocation　 __ Extra dose
__ Delayed test/　　　　 __ Wrong medication
　 treatment　　　　　　 __ Wrong dose
__ Missed test/treatment　__ Wrong time
__ Adverse reaction
__ Other:_____

disciplined or dismissed by management because of the error, it's unlikely people will voluntarily incriminate themselves or their colleagues by completing incident reports. In some instances, professional organizations may be contributing to this punitive philosophy. For example, the rule 217.19 of the Rules and Regulations relating to Professional Nurse Education, Licensure and Practice in Texas require that nurse managers maintain a record of minor incidents committed by nurses under their charge.[29] If three minor incidents involving an RN are documented within a one-year period, the facility's peer review committee must review the three minor incidents and make a determination as to whether a report to the Board of Nurse Examiners is warranted. If there is no institutional peer review committee, the nurse manager must report these minor incidents directly to the Texas Board of Nurse Examiners for further investigation and possible disciplinary action. The intent of these statutes is to identify and correct professional practice conduct that poses a risk of harm to the client. However, these and other oversight or disciplinary activities by licensing or peer review boards may continue to promulgate a philosophy of individual blame rather than continuous process improvement, causing nurses and other health care professionals to be reluctant to report errors.[30,31]

Experience has shown that when caregivers are provided protection from disciplinary actions, they are more willing to report incidents.[32,33] This phenomenon is consistent with what has been discovered by officials of the NASA Aviation Safety Reporting System and the British Airways Safety Information System. These groups have found that the following five factors are important in determining both the quantity and quality of incident reports:[34]

1. Indemnity against disciplinary proceedings (as far as it is practical)
2. Confidentiality or de-identification
3. The separation of the agency or department collecting and analyzing the reports from those bodies with the authority to institute disciplinary proceedings and impose sanctions
4. Rapid, useful, accessible, and intelligible feedback to the reporting community
5. Ease of making the report

Creating a climate of trust is an essential component of an incident-reporting system. It must also be easy for people to file reports. The

Institute for Healthcare Improvement's National Collaborative on Reducing Adverse Drug Events and Medical Errors has recommended several ways of making reporting easy for caregivers. These recommendations include establishing dial-in hotlines and instituting simplified, anonymous error-reporting mechanisms.[35]

The second challenge related to incident reporting is that the data items are not well defined or understood by the staff. For example, there must be a clear understanding of what constitutes a medication error to ensure that all such events are consistently reported. The definition of a medication error suggested by the American Society of Health-System Pharmacists reads as follows:[36]

> Any preventable event that may cause or lead to inappropriate medication use or patient harm while the medication is in the control of the health care professional, patient, or consumer. Such events may be related to professional practice, health care products, procedures and systems, including prescribing; order communication; product labeling, packaging and nomenclature; compounding; dispensing; distribution; administration; education; monitoring; and use.

This definition suggests that any error involving medication usage should be reported. However, in actual practice it is common for caregivers to raise many questions about this definition. Does this mean that the patient actually had to receive the wrong medication? Does this mean I have to report someone else's error if I discover it? Does this mean I have to complete two incident reports if the pharmacy sent the wrong drug and I gave it to the patient? Questions such as these are an indication that the definition of a reportable medication error is still not clear. The same definition problems can be found for other types of incidents. For example, if a patient is found lying unharmed on the floor, is this situation considered a fall?

Organizations should develop objective definitions of the types of incidents that must be reported. The definitions of various types of adverse events that originate from organizations such as the American Society of Health-System Pharmacists, the World Health Organization, the Joint Commission, and others should be considered when developing internal definitions. Shown in figure 2-5 are examples of various incidents and accompanying explanations that might be considered reportable in a health care organization.

Figure 2-5.   Definitions for Common Reportable Incidents

Suicide gesture

Suicidal behavior that does not meet the definition for suicide attempt

Suicide attempt

Suicidal behavior that is either medically serious or psychiatrically serious. Examples of medically serious incidents are those that result in permanent disability or disfigurement and acts that would have been lethal were it not for the intervention of another party. This would include acts that require life-saving medical interventions. A suicidal act will be considered psychiatrically serious if the patient's psychiatric condition were such that any suicidal behavior had serious implications for the patient's future care. Examples of psychiatric seriousness currently suggested by psychiatric experts include the following:

- Any suicidal behavior by a patient meeting the full DSM-III-R criteria for Major Affective Disorder
- Suicidal behavior in a substance-abusing patient with recent or impending major life disruption (e.g., marital separation, death of a loved one)
- Any suicidal behavior in a schizophrenic patient characterized by feelings of hopelessness, secondary depression, or a history of previous suicidal behavior

Suicide

Act of taking one's own life voluntarily and accidentally

Alleged patient abuse

Includes acts of physical, psychological, sexual, or verbal abuse. Employee "intent" is not a requirement for patient abuse. The patient's perception of how he or she was treated is an essential component of the determination as to whether a patient was abused. However, the fact that a patient has limited or no cognitive ability does not exclude the possibility that a patient was abused. Patient abuse may include the following components:

- Any action or behavior that conflicts with a patient's rights
- Intentional omission of patient care
- Willful violations of the privacy of a patient
- Intimidation, harassment, or ridicule of a patient
- Willful physical injury of a patient

Rape/attempted rape

Sexual assault with or without penetration

Homicide

- Death of a patient or staff caused by a patient
- Death of a patient caused by another individual

Figure 2-5.   (Continued)

Patient-on-staff abuse

- Physical injury
- Intentionally striking staff
- Permanent disability

Patient-on-patient abuse

- Patient injured by another patient
- Patient assaulted by another patient

Falls

All falls whether observed or not observed and whether or not there is injury

Blood transfusion error

Blood or blood products erroneously administered to wrong patient, therapy not ordered, wrong blood product administered, error in typing/cross-matching, with or without any reaction or evident adverse effect

Medication error

A medication error is broadly defined as a dose of medication that deviates from the physician's order as written in the patient's chart or as written on an outpatient prescription or from standard medical center procedures. Except for errors of omission, the medication dose must actually reach the patient; a wrong dose that is detected and corrected before administration to the patient is not considered a medication error. The categories of medication errors are:

- Omission error
- Wrong dose error
- Wrong rate error
- Wrong time error
- Incorrect administration technique
- Unauthorized drug error
- Wrong route error
- Wrong dosage form error
- Wrong preparation of a dose

Incorrect medications dispensed to outpatients will be considered medication errors.

It is a medication error when individual or specialized inpatient or outpatient prescriptions, including intravenous admixtures compounded by pharmacy service, do not meet all labeling requirements. In these cases, the medication does not have to be administered to the patient for it to be considered a medication error.

It is considered a medication error when the additive to the IV mixture is incorrect, be it type of medication or dosage.

Potential medication error

A medication order that requires correction by the pharmacist. The categories of potential medication errors are:

- Omissions in patient identification
- Incorrect dose, frequency, or administration route
- Other (e.g., illegible order, drug ordered for patient with known allergy, etc.)

(Continued on next page)

Figure 2-5.   (Continued)

Medication reaction

Anaphylaxis or other adverse reactions seriously affecting the well-being of a patient

Idiosyncratic reaction to blood or blood products

Reaction to blood or blood product that has been properly typed/cross-matched and administered

Surgery-related death

Includes death:

- in operating room
- in recovery room
- during induction of anesthesia
- within 48 hours of surgery

Unexpected death

Examples include the following:

- Death during or following procedures such as cardiac catheterization, biopsy, radiological procedure, or endoscopy
- Cause of death unknown
- Death reportable to local medical examiner or coroner
- Death due to previously unknown problem or diagnosis
- Death due to misadventure such as respirator malfunction, medication error, failure to diagnose, or failure to treat appropriately

Patient involved in fires

Patient:

- sets the fire
- is involved in a fire
- is burned
- is exposed to smoke of fire; i.e., smoke inhalation

Inaccurate counts in surgery

- Needles
- Sponges
- Pads

Diagnostic error

- Failure to diagnose a problem
- Failure to do proper diagnostic procedures
- Misdiagnosis

Incidents that result or may result in disability or disfigurement

Permanent disability or disfigurement or extensive corrective therapy/surgery required

Incident reports can also lack sufficient detail about the event that limits the value of aggregate data analysis. The goal of evaluating incident report data is to identify which safety-critical tasks are failing and how often these failures occur. Often, incident reports don't contain sufficient task-level information; that is, the activity that contributed to the occurrence. Without meaningful data there can be no meaningful analysis. Consider the patient incident summary report illustrated in figure 2-6. Aggregated counts are shown for the hospital nursing department as a whole and for other departments. Summary counts such as these are not focused or specific and do not reveal which safety-critical tasks are failing. At best, they serve as a global report card.

Measures of actual activities will generally be more useful than simple counts of how many times an incident occurs.[37] However, to obtain data about actual activities it is necessary to expand the data elements collected on incident reports. Figure 2-7 illustrates a sample incident report designed by Humana, Inc., for acute care facilities.[38] This report

Figure 2-6. Sample Aggregate Incident Report for a Hospital

Summary of Patient Incidents
August 1998

Nursing Services	August	Year to Date
1. Total monthly incidents	47	423
2. Incidents by classification		
A. Falls	8	72
B. Medication errors	17	237
C. Medical-clinical	9	31
D. Needle sticks	10	71
E. Other/miscellaneous	3	12

Number of Incidents in Other Departments for the Month of August

Area	Falls	Medication Errors	Medical/ Clinical	Needle Punctures	Misc.
Emergency department	1	8	0	2	1
Surgical department	0	1	0	1	0
Radiology	2	0	0	0	1
Psychiatric department	2	5	2	0	2
Laboratory	0	0	0	1	1
Pulmonary diagnostic department	0	2	0	0	0
Rehabilitation department	2	0	0	0	0

46

Figure 2-7. Occurrence Report

CONFIDENTIAL—DO NOT PHOTOCOPY • DO NOT PLACE IN MEDICAL RECORD

HUMANA

MEMBER OCCURRENCE REPORT
HU-51 (6/98)

Prepared for QA purposes or for Legal Counsel in Anticipation of Litigation

COMPLETE ALL APPLICABLE INFORMATION

PRINT OR TYPE ALL INFORMATION

MEMBER INFORMATION

NAME

ADDRESS

CITY   STATE   ZIP

DOB   SEX ☐ Female ☐ Male

PHONE #
Home: ( )   Work: ( )

SOCIAL SECURITY NUMBER

MEDICAL RECORD NUMBER

IDENTIFYING DATA—LOCATION OF OCCURRENCE

DATE OF OCCURRENCE   TIME OF OCCURRENCE   AM   PM

PROVIDER NAME

ADDRESS

CITY   STATE   ZIP

SPECIALTY

PROVIDER PHONE #
( )

HUMANA FACILITY ID# (IF APPLICABLE)

Utilize the space provided. Give a brief, factual description of occurrence to include exact location of occurrence, any injury/illness, body part affected, treatment required and reaction of involved person/witness.

☐ INJURY   ☐ ILLNESS   BODY PART (INDICATE RIGHT, LEFT, UPPER, LOWER)

DESCRIBE FACTS OF OCCURRENCE

Person(s) who witnessed or were directly involved in occurrence other than the member listed above.

NAME

ADDRESS

CITY		STATE	ZIP

PHONE #
Home: ( )   Work: ( )

SOCIAL SECURITY NUMBER

NAME

ADDRESS

CITY		STATE	ZIP

PHONE #
Home: ( )   Work: ( )

SOCIAL SECURITY NUMBER

CHECK MOST APPLICABLE CODE

CATEGORY CODES

- ☐ 101 CONFIDENTIALITY
- ☐ 102 DEATH
- ☐ 103 DISSATISFACTION/GRIEVANCE
- ☐ 104 EQUIPMENT/SHARPS/SUPPLIES
- ☐ 106 INFECTIOUS DISEASE EXPOSURE
- ☐ 107 MATERNAL/INFANT
- ☐ 108 MEDICAL RECORD
- ☐ 109 MEDICATION
- ☐ 111 N.O.S.—NOT OTHERWISE SPECIFIED
- ☐ 112 PERSONAL PROPERTY
- ☐ 113 SLIP/TRIP/FALL
- ☐ 115 THREAT/ATTACK/ALTERCATION
- ☐ 117 TOXIC/HAZARDOUS MATERIAL EXPOSURE
- ☐ 118 TREATMENT/TEST/PROCEDURE

CHECK MOST APPLICABLE CODE

CAUSE CODES

- ☐ 02 POLICY AND PROCEDURE NOT FOLLOWED
- ☐ 04 ESTABLISHED PROTOCOL NOT FOLLOWED
- ☐ 13 PERSON DEMONSTRATED UNDERSTANDING OF INSTRUCTIONS BUT DISREGARDED
- ☐ 23 UNANTICIPATED CHANGE IN MEMBER CONDITION
- ☐ 25 CARE RENDERED NOT ACCEPTABLE TO MEMBER
- ☐ 28 UNSAFE ENVIRONMENTAL CONDITION NOT CORRECTED
- ☐ 29 INATTENTION TO ACTIVITY PERFORMED
- ☐ 35 UNABLE TO CONTROL ENVIRONMENTAL CONDITION
- ☐ 37 FAILURE TO SAFEGUARD BELONGINGS
- ☐ 20 MEDICAL ORDERS/TEST RESULTS/INSTRUCTIONS ETC. NOT COMMUNICATED
- ☐ 38 NON-CREDENTIALED PROVIDER ADMINISTERED CARE TO MEMBER
- ☐ 39 NOT OTHERWISE SPECIFIED (EXPLAIN IN FACTUAL DESCRIPTION ABOVE)

COMPLETED BY	PRINT NAME	TITLE
	SIGNATURE	DATE

FORWARD TO HUMANA RISK MANAGER/DESIGNEE UPON COMPLETION

(Continued on next page)

47

Figure 2-7. (Continued)

OCCURRENCE INVESTIGATION REPORT
To Be Completed by Risk Manager/Designee

DATE OCCURRENCE REPORT RECEIVED BY RISK MANAGER	MARKET NAME/ID NUMBER

SEVERITY CODES

CHECK MOST APPLICABLE CODE

- ☐ 20 NO MEDICAL TREATMENT REQUIRED
- ☐ 21 MEDICAL TREATMENT GIVEN
- ☐ 22 EMERGENCY ROOM EVALUATION REQUIRED
- ☐ 23 HOSPITALIZATION
- ☐ 24 DEATH
- ☐ 25 NON INJURY/ILLNESS

WAS PROBABLE CLAIM FORM COMPLETED?
☐ Yes ☐ No

DOES OCCURRENCE MEET CRITERIA FOR SIGNIFICANT EVENT?
☐ Yes ☐ No

WAS MEMBER ENROLLED IN A DISEASE MANAGEMENT PROGRAM?
☐ Yes ☐ No

IF YES, LIST THE PROGRAM ONLY IF APPLICABLE TO THE OCCURRENCE

WAS A DELEGATED FUNCTION INVOLVED IN THE OCCURRENCE?
☐ Yes ☐ No

IF YES, LIST FUNCTION

COMMITTEE TO WHICH OCCURRENCE REPORTED

INVESTIGATIVE FINDINGS

RECOMMENDATIONS/PLAN OF ACTION

SIGNATURE OF RISK MANAGER/DESIGNEE	DATE

FORWARD COMPLETED OCCURRENCE REPORT TO INSURANCE RISK MANAGEMENT DEPARTMENT

includes detailed descriptions of various occurrences, incident severity, and contributing causes. The cause information could be used to create detailed reports of the actual activities that contributed to the occurrence of the incident (for example, how many times a patient was left unattended and the patient fell or how many times miscommunication of information resulted in a medication error). Instead of a mere review of the total numbers of incidents, identifying the error-producing factors that contributed to events management provides a better means of developing appropriate focused corrective actions.[39]

In an effort to standardize the details collected about medication errors in all health care facilities, the National Coordinating Council for Medication Error Reporting and Prevention (NCC MERP) of the United States Pharmacopeia has proposed a taxonomy of medication errors to be used in combination with systems analysis in recording and tracking medication errors.[40] The purpose of this taxonomy (shown in figure 2-8) is to provide a standard language and structure for medication error-related data. By gathering information at the level of detail suggested by the NCC MERP, health care facilities can begin to identify the safety-critical tasks that are not well performed and show how such failures are affecting the high-risk activity of medication usage.

The fourth problem with using incident reports as a data source for error management purposes is that not all reportable events end up getting documented. Institutions may have specific policies about what incidents to report, but studies have shown that when faced with real clinical situations, clinicians do not appear to consistently comply with those policies.[41,42] As a result much important information about errors is lost. All errors and near misses should be reported regardless of the surrounding circumstances. With this is mind, it is important to promote an atmosphere that encourages honest reporting.

There is also a belief in the risk management community that incident reports are rarely completed for truly serious events. Many professional liability carriers report that of total claims filed, only one-third ever had incident reports generated. This underreporting of serious events may be caused by staff not perceiving a problem whereas the patient does. Consider this example: A patient with a history of heart disease has a cardiac arrest on the first postoperative day. The staff feels everything was handled without error if the resuscitation is successful. From the patient's perspective, however, something went very wrong. The patient believes that the physicians and staff knew about his

Figure 2-8.   Taxonomy of Medication Errors Recommended by the National Coordinating Council for Medication Error Reporting and Prevention, United States Pharmacopeia

Preamble

This document provides a standard taxonomy of medication errors to be used in combination with systems analysis in recording and tracking of medication errors. It is not intended to assess blame. The document is not all-inclusive, but can be expanded as new issues arise. The purpose of this taxonomy is to provide a standard language and structure of medication error-related data for use in developing databases analyzing medication error reports.

Guidance is provided to assist in the application of this instrument. Please note that the taxonomy is not designed as a reporting form, but is rather a tool to categorize and analyze reports of medication errors. It is recommended that health care organizations develop systems and procedures to collect adequate information needed to analyze and report medication errors at the time the error occurs. In most cases, it should not be necessary to conduct retrospective audits to collect the needed information in order to apply this taxonomy.

The effectiveness of the taxonomy, and the resulting analysis of medication error reports, is dependent upon the amount and the quality of the data collected through medication error reports. For optimum application of the taxonomy, include as much information as possible in the instrument. However, if all the information described in the taxonomy is not collected, the information that is available should be categorized as shown in the taxonomy.

Specific Instructions

1. Note that some fields require selection from a defined list of choices and other fields require entry of free text.
2. To use the taxonomy properly, choose the most specific code available. If this level of specificity is not possible, select the code of the parent category.

10   PATIENT INFORMATION

[The purpose of this section is to:
- permit entry of an identification code that allows matching information in the taxonomy with medication error reports
- allow sorting and reporting of medication error reports (e.g., analyze medication error reports by age ranges)

For a report of Category A error (see item #31), this section can be omitted. Otherwise, complete as many of these sections as possible].

10.1   Identification Number or Initials: _____

10.2   Age—Date of Birth

10.3   Gender

10.4   Weight [may be omitted unless directly pertinent to the error (e.g., medication overdose in a pediatric patient)].

(Continued on next page)

Figure 2-8. (Continued)

20 THE EVENT

    21   <u>DATE (mmddyyyy)</u>

        [Complete as many items as possible in this section]

        21.1   Date of event

                21.1.1   Weekend

                21.1.2   Holiday

        21.2   Date of Initial Report

        21.3   Date of Follow-up Report

    22   <u>TIME</u>

        22.1   Time of Error (24 hour clock)

    23   <u>SETTING</u> (of initial error)

        [Select either one category or one subcategory, whichever provides the best known information]

        23.1   Adult Day Health Care

        23.2   Assisted Living/Board and Care

        23.3   Correctional Facility

        23.4   Emergency Rescue Unit

        23.5   Health Food Store

        23.6   Hospice

        23.7   Hospital

                23.7.1   Cardiac Step Down

                23.7.2   Central Supply

                23.7.3   Emergency Room

                23.7.4   Intensive Care Unit (ICU)

                        23.7.4.1   Cardiac ICU

                        23.7.4.2   Medical ICU

                        23.7.4.3   Neonatal ICU/Step Down (Infant Transitional)

                        23.7.4.4   Pediatric ICU

                        23.7.4.5   Surgical ICU

                23.7.5   Labor/Delivery

                23.7.6   Long Term Acute Care

                23.7.7   Nursery

                23.7.8   Nursing Unit

                23.7.9   Oncology

                23.7.10   Operating Room

                23.7.11   Outpatient

                23.7.12   Pediatrics

                23.7.13   Pharmacy

                        23.7.13.1   Inpatient

                        23.7.13.2   Outpatient

                        23.7.13.3   Nuclear

                23.7.14   Psychiatric Unit

Figure 2-8.   (Continued)

	23.7.15 Radiology
	23.7.15.1 Nuclear
	23.7.15.2 Special Procedures Area
	23.7.16 Respiratory Therapy
	23.7.17 Recovery Room (PACU)
	23.7.18 Sub-acute Care
	23.7.19 Other
23.8	Home Health Care
23.9	Mental Health Facility
23.10	Nursing Facility (Free Standing)
	23.10.1 Skilled
	23.10.2 Intermediate
	23.10.3 Pharmacy
23.11	Outpatient Facility
	23.11.1 Ambulatory Surgery
	23.11.2 Rehabilitation
	23.11.3 Urgent Care Clinic
23.12	Patient's Home/Work
23.13	Pharmacy
	23.13.1 Community
	23.13.2 Home Health Care
	23.13.3 Long Term Care
	23.13.4 Mail Service
	23.13.5 Managed Care
	23.13.6 Mental Health
	23.13.7 Nuclear
23.14	Prescriber's Office
23.15	School
23.16	Other
23.17	Unknown

24   SETTING (Where Error Perpetuated)

[Select as many settings as are applicable]

24.1	Adult Day Health Care
24.2	Assisted Living/Board and Care
24.3	Correctional Facility
24.4	Emergency Rescue Unit
24.5	Health Food Store
24.6	Hospice
24.7	Hospital
	24.7.1 Cardiac Step Down
	24.7.2 Central Supply

(Continued on next page)

Figure 2-8.   (Continued)

24.7.3	Emergency Room	
24.7.4	Intensive Care Unit (ICU)	
	24.7.4.1	Cardiac ICU
	24.7.4.2	Medical ICU
	24.7.4.3	Neonatal ICU/Step Down (Infant Transitional)
	24.7.4.4	Pediatric ICU
	24.7.4.5	Surgical ICU
24.7.5	Labor/Delivery	
24.7.6	Long Term Acute Care	
24.7.7	Nursery	
24.7.8	Nursing Unit	
24.7.9	Oncology	
24.7.10	Operating Room	
24.7.11	Outpatient	
24.7.12	Pediatrics	
24.7.13	Pharmacy	
	24.7.13.1	Inpatient
	24.7.13.2	Outpatient
	24.7.13.3	Nuclear
24.7.14	Psychiatric Unit	
24.7.15	Radiology	
	24.7.15.1	Nuclear
	24.7.15.2	Special Procedures Area
24.7.16	Respiratory Therapy	
24.7.17	Recovery Room (PACU)	
24.7.18	Sub-acute Care	
24.7.19	Other	

24.8   Home Health Care

24.9   Mental Health Facility

24.10   Nursing Facility (Free Standing)
    24.10.1   Skilled
    24.10.2   Intermediate
    24.10.3   Pharmacy

24.11   Outpatient Facility
    24.11.1   Ambulatory Surgery
    24.11.2   Rehabilitation
    24.11.3   Urgent Care Clinic

24.12   Patient's Home/Work

24.13   Pharmacy
    24.13.1   Community
    24.13.2   Home Health Care
    24.13.3   Long Term Care

Figure 2-8.   (Continued)

        24.13.4   Mail Service

        24.13.5   Managed Care

        24.13.6   Mental Health

        24.13.7   Nuclear

   24.14   Prescriber's Office

   24.15   School

   24.16   Other

   24.17   Unknown

25   DESCRIPTION OF EVENT

[This is a free text entry field. The user should provide a narrative description of the event, including how the error was perpetuated and discovered. Other relevant information should be included, such as:

- Laboratory data or tests, including dates
- Other relevant history, including preexisting medical conditions (e.g., allergies)
- Concomitant therapy
- Dates of therapy
- Indication for use (Diagnosis)
- Medical intervention(s) following the error
- Actions taken and recommendation for prevention]

30   PATIENT OUTCOME

[NCC MERP recommends that medication error information be collected and reported as soon as possible, while the information is still fresh. It is recognized that the eventual patient outcome may change from the time when the medication error initially occurs. For example, the patient may initially require hospitalization due to the error, but eventually die as a result of the error after several weeks of treatment and support in the hospital. If the patient outcome or other variables should change, the medication error information can be updated or corrected at a later time.

In selecting the patient outcome category, select the highest level severity that applies during the course of the event. For example, if a patient suffers a severe anaphylactic reaction (Category H) and requires treatment (Category F) but eventually recovers completely, the event should be coded as Category H (33.4).

Select only one of the medication error categories or subcategories, whichever best fits the error that is being reported.

   31   <u>NO ERROR</u>

        31.1   Category A

                    Circumstances or events that have the capacity to cause error

(Continued on next page)

Figure 2-8. (Continued)

32   <u>ERROR, NO HARM</u>
[Note: Harm is defined as death, or temporary or permanent impairment of body function/structure requiring intervention. Intervention may include monitoring the patient's condition, change in therapy, or active medical or surgical treatment.]

     32.1   Category B
           An error occurred but the medication did not reach the patient

     32.2   Category C (An error occurred that reaches the patient, but did not cause harm)
           32.2.1   Medication reaches the patient and is administered
           32.2.2   Medication reaches the patient but not administered

     32.3   Category D
           An error occurred that resulted in the need for increased patient monitoring, but no patient harm

33   <u>ERROR, HARM</u>
     33.1   Category E
           An error occurred that resulted in need for treatment or intervention and caused temporary patient harm

     33.2   Category F
           An error occurred that resulted in initial or prolonged hospitalization and caused temporary patient harm

     33.3   Category G
           An error occurred that resulted in permanent patient harm

     33.4   Category H
           An error occurred that resulted in a near-death event (e.g., anaphylaxis, cardiac arrest)

34   <u>ERROR, DEATH</u>
     34.1   Category I
           An error occurred that resulted in patient death.

50   PRODUCT INFORMATION—#1 [PRODUCT THAT WAS ACTUALLY (OR POTENTIALLY) GIVEN]

[Classify each medication involved in a medication error. Include the intended product for use, as well as the actual product used, if these are different. Select numbers 51-54 to code the product actually or potentially administered. Select numbers 55-59 to code the intended product, if different from the product actually administered or intended].

     51   GENERAL
           [Select and complete as many items as possible in this section].
           51.1   Name of Drug (or other products, if applicable)

Figure 2-8. (Continued)

	51.1.1	Proprietary (Trade) Name
	51.1.2	Established (Generic) Name
	51.1.3	Compounded Ingredients
51.2	Strength	
51.3	Dose, Frequency & Route	
51.4	Status	
	51.4.1	Prescription
	51.4.2	Over-the-Counter
	51.4.3	Investigational
51.5	Name of Manufacturer	
51.6	Name of Labeler or Distributor	

52   DOSAGE FORM
       [Note: This list is not all inclusive; other dosage forms not listed
       should be captured under "other". Select one item from this section]

52.1	Tablet	
	52.1.1	Extended-release
52.2	Capsule	
	52.2.1	Extended-release
52.3	Oral Liquid	
	52.3.1	Concentrate
52.4	Injectable	
52.5	Cream-Ointment-Gel-Paste	
52.6	Aerosol (spray and metered)	
52.7	Other	

53   PACKAGING—CONTAINER
       [Note that these are some examples of packaging frequently
       involved in errors. The list does not include all packaging config-
       urations available in the market place. Select one item from this
       section]

53.1	Unit Dose	
53.2	Multiple Dose Vials (Injectable)	
53.3	Single Dose Vials/Ampuls (Injectable)	
53.4	Intravenous Solutions (small and large volume parenterals)	
	53.4.1	Manufacturer Prepared
	53.4.2	Institution Prepared
53.5	Syringes	
53.6	Manufacturer Samples	
53.7	Other (Please specify)	

54   PHARMACOLOGIC-THERAPEUTIC CLASSIFICATION
       The council recommends the use of the pharmacologic-
       therapeutic classification system defined by either the American
       Society of Health-Systems Pharmacists (i.e., AHFS code) or the
       Veterans Administration (i.e., VA codes).

(Continued on next page)

Figure 2-8.   (Continued)

55	PRODUCT INFORMATION—#2 (PRODUCT THAT WAS INTENDED TO BE GIVEN)	
56	GENERAL	

[Select and complete as many items as possible in this section].

	56.1	Name
		56.1.1 Proprietary (Trade) Name
		56.1.2 Established (Generic) Name
		56.1.3 Compounded Ingredients
	56.2	Strength
	56.3	Dose, Frequency & Route
	56.4	Status
		56.4.1 Prescription
		56.4.2 Over-the-Counter
		56.4.3 Investigational
	56.5	Name of Manufacturer
	56.6	Name of Labeler or Distributor

57	DOSAGE FORM	

[Note: This list is not all inclusive; other dosage forms not listed should be captured under "other". Select one item from this section]

	57.1	Tablet
		57.1.1 Extended-release
	57.2	Capsule
		57.2.1 Extended-release
	57.3	Oral Liquid
		57.3.1 Concentrate
	57.4	Injectable
	57.5	Cream-Ointment-Gel-Paste
	57.6	Aerosol (spray and metered)
	57.7	Other

58	PACKAGING—CONTAINER	

[Note that these are some examples of packaging frequently involved in errors. The list does not include all packaging configurations available in the market place. Select one item from this section].

	58.1	Unit Dose
	58.2	Multiple Dose Vials (Injectable)
	58.3	Single Dose Vials/Ampuls (Injectable)
	58.4	Intravenous Solutions (small and large volume parenterals)
		58.4.1 Manufacturer Prepared
		58.4.2 Institution Prepared
	58.5	Syringes

Figure 2-8. (Continued)

58.6　　Manufacturer Samples
58.7　　Other (Please specify)

59　　PHARMACOLOGIC-THERAPEUTIC CLASSIFICATION
The council recommends the use of the pharmacologic-therapeutic classification system defined by either the American Society of Health-Systems Pharmacists (i.e., AHFS code) or the Veterans Administration (i.e., VA codes).

60　　PERSONNEL INVOLVED

61　Initial Error Made by
[Select one item]
61.1　　Physician
61.1.1　Intern
61.1.2　Resident
61.1.3　Practicing Physician
61.1.4　Other
61.2　　Pharmacist
61.3　　Nurse
61.3.1　Nurse Practitioner/Advanced Practice
61.3.2　Registered Nurse
61.3.3　Licensed Practical Nurse
61.3.4　Other _____
61.4　　Physician Assistant
61.5　　Dentist
61.6　　Veterinarian
61.7　　Optometrist
61.8　　Support Personnel
61.8.1　Pharmacy Technician
61.8.2　Nurses Aide
61.8.3　Medication Aide
61.8.4　Clerical
61.9　　Health Professions Student
61.9.1　Medicine
61.9.2　Pharmacy
61.9.3　Nursing
61.9.4　Other
61.10　Patient/Caregiver
61.11　Other
61.12　Unknown

62　Error Perpetuated by
[Select all that apply]
62.1　　Physician
62.1.1　Intern
62.1.2　Resident

(Continued on next page)

Figure 2-8. (Continued)

	62.1.3	Practicing Physician
	62.1.4	Other
62.2	Pharmacist	
62.3	Nurse	
	62.3.1	Nurse Practitioner/Advanced Practice
	62.3.2	Registered Nurse
	62.3.3	Licensed Practical Nurse
	62.3.4	Other _____
62.4	Physician Assistant	
62.5	Dentist	
62.6	Veterinarian	
62.7	Optometrist	
62.8	Support Personnel	
	62.8.1	Pharmacy Technician
	62.8.2	Nurses Aide
	62.8.4	Medication Aide
	62.8.5	Clerical
62.9	Health Professions Student	
	62.9.1	Medicine
	62.9.2	Pharmacy
	62.9.3	Nursing
	62.9.4	Other
62.10	Patient/Caregiver	
62.11	Other	
62.12	None	

63 Error Discovered by
[Select one item]

63.1	Physician	
	63.1.1	Intern
	63.1.2	Resident
	63.1.3	Practicing Physician
	63.1.4	Other
63.2	Pharmacist	
63.3	Nurse	
	63.3.1	Nurse Practitioner/Advanced Practice
	63.3.2	Registered Nurse
	63.3.3	Licensed Practical Nurse
	63.3.4	Other_____
63.4	Physician Assistant	
63.5	Dentist	
63.6	Veterinarian	
63.7	Optometrist	
63.8	Support Personnel	
	63.8.1	Pharmacy Technician
	63.8.2	Nurses Aide

Figure 2-8. (Continued)

	63.8.3	Medication Aide
	63.8.4	Clerical
63.9		Health Professions Student
	63.9.1	Medicine
	63.9.2	Pharmacy
	63.9.3	Nursing
	63.9.4	Other
63.10		Patient/Caregiver
63.11		Other
63.12		Unknown

70 TYPE

[Select as many items as are applicable from this section. Note: Category A errors (where only the capacity for error exists) should not be classified by Type].

70.1 Dose Omission
[The failure to administer an ordered dose to a patient before the next scheduled dose, if any. This excludes patients who refuse to take a medication or a decision not to administer.]

70.2 Improper Dose
70.2.1 Resulting in Overdosage
70.2.2 Resulting in Under dosage
70.2.3 Extra Dose

70.3 Wrong Strength/Concentration
70.4 Wrong Drug
70.5 Wrong Dosage Form
70.6 Wrong Technique (includes inappropriate crushing of tablets)
70.7 Wrong Route of Administration

Route Given		Route Intended
70.7.1	IV	Gastric
70.7.2	Intrathecal	IV
70.7.3	IV	Oral
70.7.4	IV	IM
70.7.5	IM	IV
70.7.6	Other	

70.8 Wrong Rate
70.8.1 Too fast
70.8.2 Too slow

70.9 Wrong Duration
70.10 Wrong Time
[Administration outside a predefined time interval from its scheduled administration time, as defined by each health care facility]
70.11 Wrong Patient

(Continued on next page)

Figure 2-8. (Continued)

70.12   Monitoring Error (includes Contraindicated Drugs)
    70.12.1   Drug-Drug Interaction
    70.12.2   Drug-Food/Nutrient Interaction
    70.12.3   Documented Allergy
    70.12.4   Drug-Disease Interaction
    70.12.5   Clinical (e.g., blood glucose, prothrombin, blood pressure,)
70.13   Deteriorated Drug Error (Dispensing drug which has expired)
70.14   Other
    [Any medication error that does not fall into one of the above]

80   CAUSES

[Indicate the reported causes of the medication error, as stated by the perspective of the reporter of the incident. Select as many causes as are applicable from each section]

81   <u>COMMUNICATION</u>
    81.1   Verbal miscommunication
    81.2   Written miscommunication
        81.2.1   Illegible handwriting
        81.2.2   Abbreviations
        81.2.3   Non-metric units of measurement (e.g., apothecary)
        81.2.4   Trailing Zero
        81.2.5   Leading Zero
        81.2.6   Decimal Point
        81.2.7   Misread or Didn't Read
    81.3   Misinterpretation of the order

83   <u>NAME CONFUSION</u>
    83.1   Proprietary (Trade) Name Confusion
        83.1.1   Suffix confusion
        83.1.2   Prefix confusion
        83.1.3   Sound-alike to another trade name
        83.1.4   Sound-alike to an established (generic) name
        83.1.5   Look-alike to another trade name
        83.1.6   Look-alike to an established name
        83.1.7   Appears to be misleading
        83.1.8   Confusion with Over-the-Counter "Family Trade Names"
    83.2   Established (Generic) Name Confusion
        83.2.1   Sound-alike to another established name
        83.2.2   Sound-alike to a trade name
        83.2.3   Look-alike to another established name
        83.2.4   Look-alike to a trade name

Figure 2-8. **(Continued)**

85	LABELING	
	85.1	Immediate Container Labels of Product—Manufacturer, Distributor or Repackager
		85.1.1 Looks too similar to another manufacturer
		85.1.2 Looks too similar within the same company's product line.
		85.1.3 Appears to be inaccurate or incomplete
		85.1.4 Appears to be misleading or confusing
		85.1.5 Distracting Symbols or Logo
	85.2	Labels of Dispensed Product—Practitioner
		85.2.1 Wrong Directions
		85.2.2 Incomplete Directions (including lack of ancillary labels)
		85.2.3 Wrong Drug Name
		85.2.4 Wrong Drug Strength
		85.2.5 Wrong Patient
		85.2.6 Other
	85.3	Carton Labeling of Product—Manufacturer, Distributor or Repackager
		85.3.1 Looks too similar to another manufacturer
		85.3.2 Looks too similar within the same company's product line.
		85.3.3 Appears to be inaccurate
		85.3.4 Appears to be misleading
		85.3.5 Distracting Symbols or Logo
	85.4	Package Insert
		85.4.1 Appears to be inaccurate
		85.4.2 Appears to be misleading
		85.4.3 Other
	85.5	Electronic Reference Material
		85.5.1 Inaccurate
		85.5.2 Unclear or inconsistent
		85.5.3 Omission of data
		85.5.4 Outdated
		85.5.5 Unavailable
	85.6	Printed Reference Material
		85.6.1 Inaccurate
		85.6.2 Unclear or inconsistent
		85.6.3 Omission of data
		85.6.4 Unavailable
	85.7	Advertising
		85.7.1 Error or error potential associated with the commercial advertising of a product.

(Continued on next page)

Figure 2-8. (Continued)

87 <u>HUMAN FACTORS</u>
    87.1   Knowledge Deficit
    87.2   Performance Deficit
    87.3   Miscalculation of Dosage or Infusion Rate
    87.4   Computer Error
        87.4.1   Incorrect selection from a list by computer operator
        87.4.2   Incorrect programming into the database
        87.4.3   Inadequate screening for allergies, interactions, etc.
    87.5   Error in Stocking/Restocking/Cart Filling
    87.6   Drug Preparation Error
        87.6.1   Failure to activate delivery system
        87.6.2   Wrong Diluent
        87.6.3   Wrong Amount of Diluent
        87.6.4   Wrong amount of active ingredient added to the final product
        87.6.5   Wrong drug added
    87.7   Transcription Error
        87.7.1   Original to Paper/Carbon paper
        87.7.2   Original to Computer
        87.7.3   Original to Facsimile
        87.7.4   Recopying MAR
    87.8   Stress (high volume workload, etc.)
        87.9   Fatigue/Lack of Sleep
        87.10   Confrontational or intimidating behavior

89 <u>PACKAGING/DESIGN</u>
    89.1   Inappropriate Packaging or Design
    89.2   Dosage Form (Tablet/Capsule) Confusion:
        89.2.1   Confusion due to similarity in color, shape, and/or size to another product.
        89.2.2   Confusion due to similarity in color, shape, and/or size of the same product but different strength.
    89.3   Devices
        89.3.1   Malfunction
        89.3.2   Wrong Device Selected (e.g., TB syringe used instead of Insulin syringe)
        89.3.3   Adapters (e.g., Parenteral vs Enteral)
        89.3.4   Automated Distribution/Vending Systems
        89.3.5   Automated Counting Machines

Figure 2-8.   (Continued)

	89.3.6	Automated Compounders
	89.3.7	Oral Measuring Devices (e.g., syringes, cups, spoons)
	89.3.8	Infusion (PCA, Infusion pumps)

90   CONTRIBUTING FACTORS (SYSTEMS RELATED)

[Select as many items as are applicable from this section].

90.1   Lighting
90.2   Noise Level
90.3   Frequent Interruptions and distractions
90.4   Training
90.5   Staffing
90.6   Lack of availability of health care professional
    90.6.1   Medical
    90.6.2   Other Allied Health Care Professional
    90.6.3   Pharmacy
    90.6.4   Nursing
    90.6.5   Other
90.7   Assignment or placement of a health care provider or inexperienced personnel
90.8   System for Covering Patient Care (e.g., floating personnel, agency coverage)
    90.8.1   Medical
    90.8.2   Other Allied Health Care Professional
    90.8.3   Pharmacy
    90.8.4   Nursing
    90.8.5   Other
90.9   Policies and procedures
90.10   Communication systems between health care practitioners
90.11   Patient counseling
90.12   Floor Stock
90.13   Pre-printed medication orders
90.14   Other

predisposing cardiac problems and should have taken appropriate precautions. Such differences in perception can cause the patient to initiate legal action, and yet no incident report of the event is completed by the staff.

In addition, injuries that evolve over a period of time (for example, deterioration in condition, neurological impairment, vascular compromise, and so on) are generally not reported because there may not be one particular point in time when something actually happened to cause the injury. Therefore, an incident report is not completed.

Even in the best of situations and environments, it is unlikely incident reports will ever be the sole data source for error prevention performance measurement. The information gleaned from incident reports will need to be supplemented by data obtained from other sources.

Administrative Data

Administrative data are another source of performance measurement information, particularly malpractice claims and billing data. Malpractice claims information can provide a wealth of information about potentially preventable clinical and system errors that lead to undesirable patient outcomes.[43] However, claims data are not without pitfalls and weaknesses. Many claims are filed in the absence of actual clinical errors. Plus (thankfully) the number of actual claims that are filed is small, making aggregate analyses suspect. Regardless, some people have suggested that claims data can be useful in determining types of mistakes made in patient care and for suggesting changes that need to be made.[44] Detailed claims investigation reports prepared by the risk management department may stimulate further inquiry and suggest solutions to some types of problems.

The organization's billing database, which typically contains information such as patient demographics, codes that identify diagnoses and procedures performed, and charges billed to payers, is another data source. This database can provide the data elements necessary for the denominators of some patient safety-related performance measurements (such as number of discharges, number of deaths, and so on). The coded diagnosis and procedure data may also be useful in identifying instances of iatrogenic events. For example, the E-codes contained in the International Classification of Diseases, Ninth Revision (ICD-9), have been used by researchers in Australia to identify adverse events in Australian hospitals.[45] Some of the diagnosis codes in the International Classification of Diseases, Ninth Revision, Clinical Modification (ICD-9-CM) used in the United States represent complications or comorbidities. Listed in table 2-2 are examples of diagnosis codes for fetal complications and birth injuries.[46] A simple count of these ICD-9-CM codes is not an absolute measure of adverse events; however, the codes could be used for screening purposes.[47] Further analysis of the cases to which these codes apply would be necessary to determine if inappropriate caregiver actions contributed to these conditions.

Another problem with the use of many diagnosis and procedure codes is that the data do not typically indicate when the event occurred. Without knowledge of the timing, one cannot determine whether a condition (such as decubitus ulcer) was present when the patient was admitted to the facility or arose later, possibly as a result of poor-quality care. Researchers at Brigham and Women's Hospital in Boston found that even the most sensitive screens applied to billing data could detect just 47 percent of adverse events, and yet these researchers suggested that the cost of the chart reviews necessary to find a higher number of such events might be prohibitive.[48]

Table 2-2.   ICD-9-CM Codes for Fetal Complications/Birth Injuries

ICD-9-CM Code	Description
767.0	Subdural and Cerebral Hemorrhage at Birth
767.1	Injuries to Scalp
767.2	Fracture of Clavicle
767.3	Other Injuries to Skeleton
767.4	Injury to Spine and Spinal Column
767.5	Facial Nerve Injury
767.6	Injury to Brachial Plexus
767.7	Other Cranial and Peripheral Nerve Injuries
767.8	Other Specified Birth Trauma
767.9	Birth Trauma, Unspecified
768.2	Fetal Distress before Onset of Labor in Live Born Infant
768.5	Severe Birth Asphyxia
779.0	Convulsions in Newborn
779.1	Other Unspecified Cerebral Irritability
779.2	Cerebral Depression, Coma, or Other Abnormal Cerebral Signs
779.4	Drug Reactions and Intoxications Specific to Newborns

Administrative databases that contain primarily billing information are of limited value in providing risk-related performance measurement data. Gaps in clinical information and the billing context may compromise the facility's ability to derive valid patient incident and outcome data from administrative data. The data provide insufficient clinical information, especially with regard to errors of omission and commission. However, the growing availability of electronic clinical information is changing the nature of administrative data and strengthening its usefulness as a source for safety-related performance measures. Examples of these new administrative databases are summarized below.

Skilled nursing facilities (SNFs) are required to conduct comprehensive and standardized assessment of each Medicare and Medicaid resident's functional capacity and health status. This resident assessment database (known as the Minimum Data Set, or MDS) is an example of a more comprehensive administrative data source. By comparing initial and subsequent assessment data, a facility can identify residents who have a significant change in health status. According to the Health Care Financing Administration, any decline in a resident's status that will not normally resolve itself without intervention by staff or by implementing standard disease-related clinical interventions should prompt an interdisciplinary review and/or revision of the resident's care plan.[49] In rare instances, the decline in a resident's status may be due to an untoward incident or undesirable situation (for example, medication error, fall, inadequate hygiene, and so on). This information can be gathered and documented in the SNF administrative database at the time of the resident's comprehensive assessment.

The Outcome and Assessment Information Set (OASIS) being used by home health agencies is similar to the MDS. Clients are assessed on admission and at regular intervals until discharge. The OASIS data allow home health agencies to measure individual client outcomes and identify opportunities to improve agency performance and client satisfaction.[50] This administrative database can also be a source of patient safety-related performance data for measures such as the following:

- Hospital readmission rates
- Percent of clients who fail to meet expected outcomes for various conditions
- Emergency department visit rates

- Percent of clients with history of unsafe walking/falling who are not referred for physical therapy assessment
- Percent of clients with no reported safety hazards in their home who experience a hazard-related accident
- Percent of clients developing surgical wound infections

A number of inpatient and ambulatory providers are creating computerized point-of-care documentation systems that contain fields for capturing quality-related data. One such group is Swedish Family Medicine in Seattle, Washington.[51] A computer-generated Patient Encounter Worksheet is placed in the patient's record at the time of each clinic visit. This multipurpose form has sections in which information that is already known about the patient (such as health risk factors) and health maintenance recommendations are displayed. In addition, there is a section labeled "outcome screens" where caregivers can record outcomes of care. The outcome screen section is illustrated in figure 2-9. Any physician, nurse, or office staff member can record an adverse outcome in the outcome screen section. When an adverse outcome is selected, the case is flagged for discussion at the clinic's monthly morbidity and mortality conference. In addition, the outcome data as well as other data items on the Patient Encounter Worksheet are used to create aggregate measurement reports that the physicians use to monitor performance. For example, the health maintenance data are used to monitor the safety-critical task of childhood immunizations, a process that has been steadily improving at Swedish Family Medicine as shown by the run chart in figure 2-10.

Patient Records

One of the most costly sources of performance measurement data may be patient records. In closed chart reviews of 3,137 cases conducted by the Brigham and Women's Hospital, researchers reported $13 per case review costs. Of all admissions, 341 (11 percent) were judged to include an adverse event, which translated into a cost of $116 for every discovered adverse event.[52] The cost of retrospective record review can be significantly reduced if the activity is combined with other chart analysis activities. For example, at the University Neuropsychiatric Institute in Salt Lake City, coders in the health information management department

Figure 2-9.   Patient Encounter Worksheet

01. _____ Visit not of quality assurance significance
02. _____ Hospital admit for adverse patient occurrence (APO)
03. _____ Return to clinic/emergency department for APO
04. _____ Unplanned surgical outcome
05. _____ Infectious complication
06. _____ Patient death
07. _____ Clinic-incurred incident
08. _____ Patient dissatisfaction
09. _____ Error—blood product
10. _____ Error—medication
11. _____ Error—test follow-up
12. _____ Drug reaction
13. _____ Record documentation deficiency
14. _____ Continuity/preventive care deficiency
15. _____ Delay in diagnosis
16. _____ Delay in consultation
17. _____ Other: _____

Patient Encounter Worksheet of the Quality Care Program software system at Swedish Family Medicine, Seattle, WA. Source: Lee A. Norman and Philip A. Hardin. "Computer-Assisted Outcomes Management in the Ambulatory Care Setting," in Patrice A. Spath, ed., *Medical Effectiveness and Outcomes Management: Issues, Methods, and Case Studies* (Chicago: American Hospital Publishing, Inc., 1996), p. 315. Reprinted with permission.

help the pharmacy department identify suspected adverse drug reactions (ADRs) after patients are discharged. The following process is used:[53]

1. When coding the patient's medical record, the coders review all physician notes and the discharge summary to identify possible ADRs. The coder looks for
    a. a decrease in the patient's medication that was not apparently related to the patient's diagnosis;
    b. discontinuation of the patient's medication that was not apparently related to the patient's diagnosis; and
    c. laboratory studies ordered following an apparent medication reaction.
2. Any suspected ADRs found by the coder are added to a log maintained for the pharmacy department. Each entry includes patient name, medical record number, date of discharge, and area of the chart where pharmacists should look for information about the possible ADR.

Figure 2-10.   Percentage of Children Overdue for Routine Immunizations at Quarterly Intervals (July 1993 to April 1994)

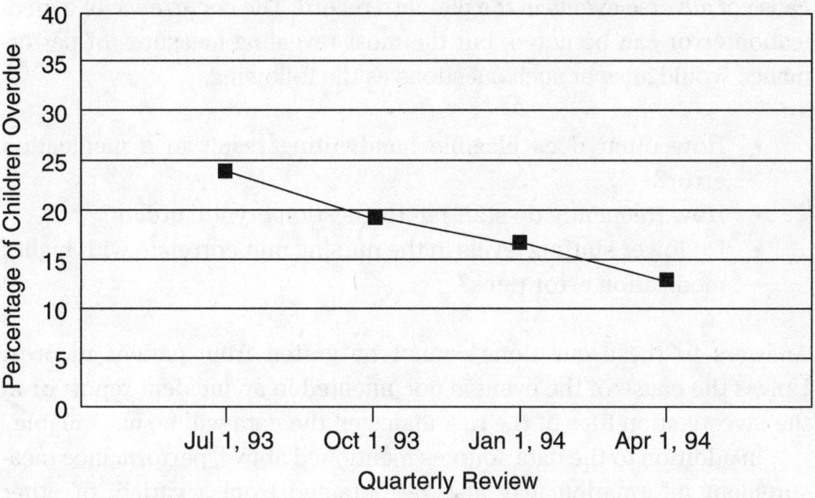

Swedish Family Medicine, Seattle, WA. Source: Lee A. Norman and Philip A. Hardin. "Computer-Assisted Outcomes Management in the Ambulatory Care Setting," in Patrice A. Spath, ed., *Medical Effectiveness and Outcomes Management: Issues, Methods, and Case Studies* (Chicago: American Hospital Publishing, Inc., 1996), p. 317. Reprinted with permission.

3. The cases identified by this process are reviewed by pharma-
    cists. All actual ADRs are confirmed by the pharmacy.

Because the coders in the health information management department at the Neuropsychiatric Institute are already reading the patient's
record to identify codable diagnoses and procedures, the cost of the
additional review for possible ADRs is negligible. When provided with
explicit criteria, health information management professionals can reliably identify the cases that need more in-depth analysis by clinicians.[54]
One of the pitfalls of using patient records to identify the underlying
system issues surrounding adverse events is the lack of detail. For example, if a patient receives the wrong dose of a medication, the nurse's
notes may read something like, "Patient received 10 mg instead of the 5
mg that was ordered by the physician." Information about the patient's
response will also be recorded by the nurse. What is likely to be missing
from the chart is the cause of the event. Perhaps the doctor's handwriting was unclear, and because of the urgency of the situation, the staff did

not clarify the order with the physician. To protect such information from disclosure, caregivers are rightfully urged not to document the cause of adverse events in the patient's record. The occurrence of a medication error can be noted, but the most revealing measures of performance would answer such questions as the following:

- How often does illegible handwriting result in a medication error?
- How frequently do staff fail to question cryptic orders?
- Do lower staffing levels in the nursing unit correlate with higher medication error rates?

Answers to these questions cannot be gotten from patient records. Unless the cause of the event is documented in an incident report or in the investigation files of the risk manager, the data will be unavailable.

In addition to the data sources mentioned above, performance measurement information may also be obtained from a variety of other sources, such as patient and staff surveys, patient care logs (for example, operating room, emergency department, and clinic encounters), and special computerized databases (such as pharmacy and laboratory data). When planning the data collection strategy, evaluate existing data sources to determine where the information necessary to create each performance measure can be found.[55] First determine if the necessary data are accessible in an existing information system. If they are, then check to be sure the data definitions are consistent with what you need for the measure. Although it may seem as if every possible data element is now being gathered, there may be times when the data needed to calculate a particularly important measure are not readily available and new data sources will need to be developed.

ANALYZE MEASUREMENT RESULTS

An effective error management strategy requires that performance measurement results be processed and presented in meaningful ways to clinical and administrative staff. Individual departments should receive their own measurement reports; however, the organization should also identify a leadership group that is responsible for overseeing error management activities throughout the facility. This may be the quality council, risk management committee, or another specially appointed ad hoc committee. In the context of this chapter, this group will be called the error management committee. This group should receive organizationwide risk-related performance measurement results for analysis. To create this aggregate report, start by gathering together all the measures that relate to patient safety so they can be merged into one report. Next use data analysis techniques to identify the early warning signs of safety-related problems that require immediate investigation and action.

Compile Risk-Related Measures

Health care organizations commonly create department- or service-specific performance reports, each of which include some risk-related measurement data. For example, hospital nursing units could be measuring compliance with medication administration protocols while the emergency department might be reporting the percentage of charts lacking information about patients' home medications. Since the data for these measures are collected and reported separately, no one individual or group has a comprehensive picture of how well the entire organization is doing relative to the high-risk activity of medication usage.

To gain a thorough understanding of how well caregivers are performing high-risk processes, the safety-related performance measures from each department-specific report should be duplicated onto an error management summary. This summary report would include the results of every department's measures of performance for high-risk processes plus relevant outcome measures. Combining these data into one report can make it easier to identify relationships between process breakdowns and outcomes. For example, there may be a correlation between surgical site infections and missed or delayed doses of antibiotics. However, this correlation will be difficult (if not impossible) to see if the measurement data appear on separate reports. Combining all risk-related measures into one organizationwide report can also help to ensure that small problems that are prevalent in more than one department are discovered and corrected. For example, nurses in the operating room may be experiencing periodic problems with broken equipment. While this is an annoyance, the number of incidents may never reach the threshold for further investigation. Home health nurses may also be having the same problems, but they don't take any action either as the number of incidents is so small. Unless one individual or group can see that the same equipment-related problems are occurring in several service areas, this circumstance will likely go uncorrected and could lead to serious patient injury.

Start the process of aggregating performance data about high-risk processes by listing each department's current patient safety-relevant process and outcome measures. Have the error management committee review the list to be sure all important functions are covered as well as are high-risk safety-critical tasks. It may be necessary to add some new measures. Once the inventory of measures is finalized, the next step is to capture the numbers from each department's report and merge them into an organizationwide error management report. The measures on this report can be sorted into categories, such as the important patient care functions identified by the Joint Commission's accreditation standards. The report shown in table 2-3 illustrates this reporting technique. Also shown is the portion of a hospital's error management report for the function of medication usage. Included on the report is a quarter-by-quarter summary of all medication-related measurement results that have been collected throughout the organization. Similar reports can be created for each major patient care function.

Use Data Analysis Techniques

Combining all measures into one report makes it easier for the error management committee to detect significant undesirable trends. Before taking action on these trends, it is important for the committee to consider the strengths and weaknesses of the data. This step allows for the identification of misinformation that might bias the analysis. Misinformation is information that is incorrect because of such factors as misinterpretation, improper recording, underreporting, and data collection mistakes.

The biggest problem with safety-related data is reporting inconsistencies. If people are punished when they report high error rates, they will start reporting lower rates regardless of the actual number of errors. Gross underreporting of medication errors through incident reports has been widely documented. In one study, 36 errors were reported via incident reports for one year, although results of a direct

Table 2-3. Error Management Report for the High-Risk Activity of Medication Usage

General Measures	4/1/98–6/30/98	7/1/98–9/30/98	10/1/98–12/31/98	1/1/99–3/31/99
Number of medication errors per 100 doses administered	3	1.4	2.1	4.3
Percent attributed to transcription errors	35%	22%	23%	15%
Percent attributed to noncompliance with established protocol	20%	15%	21%	18%
Percent attributed to miscalculation dosage/amounts/rate	13%	35%	12%	31%
Percent attributed to incorrect dispensing by pharmacy	9%	3%	8%	4%
Percent attributed to unclear/inappropriate MD order	2%	9%	12%	11%
Percent attributed to lack of response to request for needed assistance	10%	7%	13%	18%
Percent attributed to other/miscellaneous causes	11%	9%	11%	3%
Number of medication errors resulting in serious patient injury or death	0	1	0	2
Number of medication errors resulting in the need for additional medical treatment or extended hospital stay	2	1	2	4
Percent of patients developing adverse drug reaction	.6%	1.2%	.3%	.9%
Measures of Safety-Critical Activities	185	127	141	157
Percent of charts with patient's allergies noted prior to administration of antiarrhythmic medications	89%	90%	91%	88%
Percent of cases in which titration of IV Pitocin was done per hospital policy	85%	88%	88%	99%
Percent of patient medication profiles (in pharmacy) that correspond to physician's orders	97%	98%	100%	100%
Percent of benzodiazepine doses correct for patient age and/or condition	62%	84%	98%	100%
Percent of IV antibiotics administered within 1 hour of physician's order (medicine service)	83%	84%	78%	83%
Average thrombolytic therapy "door to needle" time (minutes)	45 min	76 min	69 min	48 min
Percent of patients reporting <5 on a pain scale of 1–10 on postop day 1 (surgery service)	72%	80%	75%	78%

observation sample suggested that 51,200 errors (or 1,422 times as many) may have occurred during the same year.[56] Because of these reporting discrepancies, it may be difficult to know how to react to performance measure results. High error rates may be an indicator of good detection and reporting by health care professionals, whereas low rates may be due to either lack of reporting or highly successful error prevention tactics.[57]

Not all risk-related performance measures will be affected by reporting inconsistencies. Generally, measures that rely on data that are voluntarily reported tend to be less reliable than data obtained through standardized patient record reviews, database queries, or observational studies. Therefore, accuracy may be judged differently for different types of information and can involve cross-checking information between reports; verifying numbers with knowledgeable respondents; or assessing the plausibility, detail, documentation, consistency, and overall "ring of truth."[58] If the data are not considered to be reasonably accurate, the error management committee should concentrate organizational efforts on improving the quality of the information. In some organizations, getting good numbers is the most important first step in the error management initiative.

It is not the intent of this chapter to address each and every analysis method that can be used to evaluate performance data. Methods range from fairly simple to fairly complicated. What is presented in this section is a very brief discussion of how to evaluate the fluctuations in performance data that will naturally occur from month to month. What the error management committee must determine is whether or not changes in the data represent random fluctuations in the process or if the changes represent an important signal that must be acted on.

The simplest tool that allows for identifying trends in performance measurement data is the run chart. This chart displays the data in the time order that they were collected. The run chart is constructed so that time is displayed on the horizontal axis and increases as you move to the right. The measurement data are plotted on the vertical axis. Figure 2-11 provides an example of a run chart showing the percentage of reported patient incidents that did not result in discomfort, infection, pain, or harm to the patient. The mean of the values is plotted as a horizontal line across the graph. This mean line helps the error management committee detect patterns and trends. A pattern is formed when points on the run chart consistently "move" around the mean line in the same repetitive fashion (as shown in the graph). A trend is present when successive points on the run chart show either a consistent increase in value or decrease in value. Generally seven or more points all going up or all going down are considered a trend.[59]

Measurement data can also be analyzed using statistical process control by plotting the data on a control chart such as the prototype illustrated in figure 2-12. A control chart includes the following:

- The performance measurement data
- An average (or center) line set at the mean (arithmetic average) of the data
- An upper control limit set at the mean plus three standard deviations
- A lower control limit set at the mean minus three standard deviations

A control chart is useful for determining if measurement results are attributable to common cause variation (random fluctuations in the process) or if the results indicate that special cause variation (something unusual in the process) is happening. Wheeler and Chambers provide an excellent reference for determining the correct approach for handling variation in most types of control charts.[60] In general, they suggest an estimate of the standard deviation be computed and then control limits established at three standard deviations above (the upper

Figure 2-11.   Percentage of Patient Incidents That Did Not Result in Discomfort, Infection, Pain, or Harm to the Patient

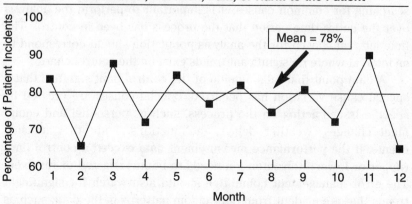

Figure 2-12. Control Chart Prototype

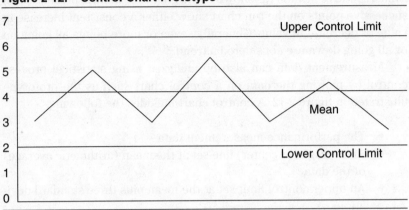

control limit) and below (the lower control limit) the mean. Common causes of variation produce data points on a control chart that over time all fall inside the control limits. In this situation, no statistically significant trend is said to exist. The performance data do vary from point to point, but the fluctuations are due to random variation in the process.

If the performance data remain within control limits for 25 data points, the process is said to be "in control." To improve an "in control" process, the error management committee must examine all of the process information over the time period the process has been stable. Improvement will hinge on determining the error-producing factors that have been acting on the process over this time and changing the process to remove or mitigate the sources of common cause variation.[61] In searching for common causes, it is important to perform the analysis over the entire time period that the process has been in control. The time interval chosen for the analysis population should correspond to an interval where no significant trends exist on the control chart.

A data point that falls outside of the control limit signifies that a special cause variation has occurred. Special causes are created by specific issues acting on the process, such as personnel and equipment changes, weather delays, malfunctions, and other unusual events. If the performance measurement data exceed a control limit (upper or lower), this situation needs to be investigated or resolved. The error management committee should also watch for significant trends that are evident from nonrandom patterns in the data, such as the following:[62]

- Two out of three points in a row outside of two standard deviations above the average or two out of three points in a row outside of two standard deviations below the average
- Four out of five points in a row outside of one standard deviation above the average or four out of five points in a row outside of one standard deviation below the average

If one of these patterns is evident in the data over at least four complete reporting cycles, the process should be investigated for special causes. When a significant sentinel event has occurred, a formal root cause analysis should be initiated. Such a detailed analysis is important for understanding the specific event as well as being required by the standards of the Joint Commission.

By using control charts instead of run charts to plot performance measurement data, the error management committee is less likely to view data fluctuations as coming from special causes. Considerable harm will be done (and certainly no improvement will be achieved) if endless hours are expended trying to explain why the most recent datum point occurred. Only if the most recent datum point was a statistically significant change on the control chart should there be an investigation into why the datum point came in at the value it did.

Benchmarking Performance

Health care benchmarking is the continual and collaborative discipline of measuring and comparing the results of key work processes with those of the best performers.[63] The two types of benchmarking that can be used to evaluate patient safety–related measurement results are internal and competitive benchmarking. Internal benchmarking is used to compare best practices within the organization. Internal benchmarking can also refer to the comparison of current practice to previous performance. Competitive benchmarking involves comparisons between organizations. To take advantage of competitive benchmarking, the error management committee must have access to performance data and process improvement recommendations from other organizations.

Internal Benchmarking   By analyzing the performance trends shown in the run chart in figure 2-11, the error management committee is conducting one type of internal benchmarking. The group is determining if organizationwide performance over time is improving, getting worse, or staying about the same. This analysis can be particularly informative if the measurement data are plotted on a control chart with statistically derived upper and lower control limits. Performance measurement data can also be used to identify best practices in the organization. For example, one unit may be experiencing failures in a safety-critical task that are not evident in other units. Rather than merely trying to justify why the problem unit may be different, caregivers should be encouraged to share process improvement ideas among themselves. Comparisons among units within an organization can be a source of superior practice.

The biggest disadvantage to internal benchmarking is that your organization's processes may not represent industry best practices. Competitive benchmarking offers the greatest potential for breakthrough improvement.[64]

Competitive Benchmarking   Health care organizations have begun to recognize the limitations of internal benchmarking and are turning their attention to what's happening outside of their facility. For error management purposes, competitive benchmarking involves two activities: the use of comparative data to judge performance and identification of process improvements that have proven to be successful error reduction tactics in other organizations.

Comparative data about risk-related performance are available at the local, state, and national levels. Some of these data are publicly available, while other comparative databases are only accessible to project participants. The report in figure 2-13 is an example of a comparative report created by United Healthcare Corporation (UHC) of North Carolina. An individual physician's practice patterns are compared with those of his peers and UHC standards. The data for the report are gathered from billing claims. Although the purpose of the report may be to encourage appropriate utilization of services, the data also provide information about important patient care processes that, if not completed as required, could represent a liability risk for the physician. Without any valid methods for adjusting the results for differences in patient case mix, severity of illness, comorbidities, and patient preferences, the data should not be used to infer quality of clinical performance.[65] However, it may help the clinic to focus error reduction initiatives on those processes where variation appears to be greatest.

Figure 2-13.   Clinical Profile

Current Report Period Ending: 5/31/1997

Health Plan: United Healthcare of North Carolina
Physician Name: Dr. #2
Specialty: Internal Medicine
Physician ID #:   #2

Please review and contact Minnie Hale
at (910) 282-6295 if you need additional
information regarding this report.

Previous Report Period Ending:

Measure includes
claims for 1 year

Use of ACE Inhibitor
drug therapy among
patients with CHF

	Your Rate		Peer Group Norm	UHC Standard
	Current	Previous		
	N/A	N/A	50%	N/A
No. Patients	0 of 0	0 of 0		

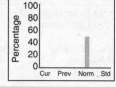

Measure includes
claims for 2 years

Use of beta blockers
following acute
myocardial infarction

	Your Rate		Peer Group Norm	UHC Standard
	Current	Previous		
	N/A	N/A	50%	N/A
No. Patients	0 of 0	0 of 0		

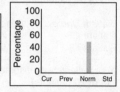

Measure includes
claims for 1 year

Use of anticoagulants
among patients with
atrial fibrillation

	Your Rate		Peer Group Norm	UHC Standard
	Current	Previous		
	N/A	N/A	0%	N/A
No. Patients	0 of 0	0 of 0		

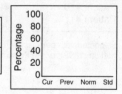

Measure includes
claims for 1 year

Potassium screening
among patients
on diuretics

	Your Rate		Peer Group Norm	UHC Standard
	Current	Previous		
	58%	N/A	60%	N/A
No. Patients	30 of 52	0 of 0		

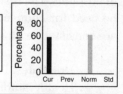

Measure includes
claims for 2 years

Biannual rate of
mammograms
among women
(age = 52–64 yrs)

	Your Rate		Peer Group Norm	UHC Standard
	Current	Previous		
	80%	N/A	77%	N/A
No. Patients	66 of 82	0 of 0		

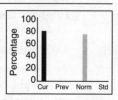

(Continued on next page)

Figure 2-13. **(Continued)**

Measure includes claims for 1 year Glycated hemoglobin screening (at least one) among diabetic patients (age > 16 yrs)	Your Rate		Peer Group Norm	UHC Standard
	Current	Previous		
	30%	N/A	60%	N/A
No. Patients	6 of 20	0 of 0		

Your patients on diuretics who may not be receiving potassium level screening are:
(22 of 82 patients)

Patient Name	Patient ID	Gender	Date of Birth	Approximate Date of the Event
Patient #6	#6	M	05/15/1956	
Patient #7	#7	F	07/22/1928	

Your patients who may not have received a biannual mammogram are:
(16 of 82 patients)

Patient Name	Patient ID	Gender	Date of Birth	Approximate Date of the Event
Patient #8	#8	F	01/10/1945	
Patient #9	#9	F	04/21/1941	

Your patients with diabetes who may not be receiving glycated hemoglobin screening are:
(14 of 20 patients)

Patient Name	Patient ID	Gender	Date of Birth	Approximate Date of the Event
Patient #10	#10	F	01/21/1947	
Patient #11	#11	F	03/13/1957	

Reprinted with permission from *Data Strategies & Benchmarks* (Atlanta, GA: National Health Information, 1998), p. 14. For subscription information, call 800-597-6300 or visit www.nhionline.net.

A number of studies have looked at the incidence of adverse events in hospitals. The results of these studies, such as those listed below, can be used for comparative purposes if the researchers' data definitions are consistent with those of your organization.

- Drs. Bates, Petrycki, and Leape of the Harvard School of Public Health studied drug-related adverse events (AEs) in 2,967 patient days over a 36-day period in adults on 7 units at Boston's Brigham and Women's Hospital. They identified 27 drug-related AEs in the 424 admissions, for a rate of 11 drug-related AEs per 1,000 patient days.[66]
- An analysis of medication error studies in approximately 40 hospitals and nursing homes in the United States and Canada covering the period from 1962 to 1987 showed that facilities'

medication error rates ranged from a high of 20.6 percent to a low of 1.6 percent when wrong timing errors were excluded. When wrong timing errors were included, the range was 42.9 percent to 4.4 percent.[67]

- Of 1,047 patient records examined from three units of a large, urban teaching hospital affiliated with a university, 185 (17.7 percent) of the patients had at least one serious adverse event.[68]

- During 1990, about 2 percent ($n = 819$) of 35,000 of the inpatients at Massachusetts General Hospital in Boston were reported to have slipped or fallen while hospitalized. Thirty-five percent fell from beds, 25 percent while walking, 15 percent from chairs, and 3 percent from equipment. Twenty-two percent of falls were unwitnessed. Most patients fell in their rooms (76 percent), and the remainder in the bathroom (14 percent), hallways (6 percent), or other locations (4 percent).[69]

- For the completed years of 1994 to 1996, a total of 262 cases were submitted to the Pediatric Cardiac Arrest Registry from participating institutions administering approximately 750,000 anesthetics. The cardiac arrest or death rate from this period was approximately 2.8 per 10,000 anesthetics. Twenty-two percent of arrests occurred during induction and 67 percent during maintenance. Thirty-one percent were emergency cases, and 16 percent were for procedures scheduled on an outpatient basis. Death within 24 hours of arrest was the final outcome for 43 percent of cases and death at 1 to 24 days following cardiac arrest for an additional 4 percent. Forty-two percent suffered no discernible injury, while 6 percent suffered a temporary injury that included an increase in level of care (following resuscitation) or delay in recovery. Four percent had injuries that were considered permanent.[70]

Databases that rely on voluntary reporting of adverse events are at highest risk of being inaccurate even when reporting is mandated by state or federal regulations. For example, hospitals have been alleged to underreport adverse actions taken against physicians to the National Practitioner Data Bank, a nationwide database that allows authorities, hospitals, and insurers in each state to keep track of problem practitioners. According to a study done by the Regional (Boston) Inspector General for Evaluation and Inspections, Office of the Inspector General,

Department of Health and Human Services, from September 1, 1990, to December 31, 1993, about 75 percent of all hospitals in the United States never reported an adverse action to the Data Bank. The author of this study suggested that it is "highly unlikely" that these minimal levels of reporting exist because there are so few practitioners with sufficient serious performance problems.[71] He suggested that one cause of the low numbers could be that hospitals are simply not reporting adverse actions.

In 1997 the Public Advocate's Office for the City of New York conducted a study of the reliability of adverse incident data reported by hospitals in New York State.[72] Since 1995, hospital administrators have been required to report patient events to the New York State Department of Health (DoH). After reviewing the data for the period July 1, 1995, through June 30, 1996, the Public Advocate's Office suggested that many hospitals were reporting only a fraction of the events that actually occur. The main contributors to underreporting were felt to be the honor system and the DoH's failure to enforce reporting requirements. A replacement reporting system, the New York Patient Occurrence Reporting and Tracking System (NYPORTS), went into effect in mid-1998. It is hoped that clearer definitions of what is and what is not reportable ("includes" and "excludes" lists) will improve reporting, although as of April 1998 the Public Advocate's Office believed that the definitions still left too much room for interpretation by individual facilities.[73]

It may be difficult for a health care organization to ever answer the question, Are we in the ballpark? when it comes to the incidence of adverse patient events. Although the number of comparative databases appears to be growing, they still lack consistency and precision. The total numbers are suspect because of the nature of voluntary reporting. There are inaccuracy problems related to differing definitions, lack of data-quality controls, and limited capacity to account for differences in patient populations. At the present time, blind use of comparative data to benchmark error management performance and establish new targets can easily lead to erroneous conclusions and inappropriate actions.

Dr. Charles Billings, who was involved in the design and implementation of NASA's Aviation Safety Reporting System (ASRS), suggests that counting voluntarily reported incidents is a waste of time.[74] The benefit of the ASRS has been in capturing and disseminating information about the sequence of events and error-producing factors surrounding airline incidents, not merely reporting prevalence data. In health care, is it really necessary to know the exact number of adverse events that occur? Billings suggests that it is more important to recognize that there are repeated mishaps involving the same drugs (for example, potassium chloride and lidocaine) or the same tasks (such as care of restrained patients) and that improvements are needed.

An example of such a mishap database is the medical device–related events database maintained by the Food and Drug Administration (FDA). The Safe Medical Devices Act of 1990 and the Medical Device Amendments of 1992 require that any "device user facility" report certain types of medical device–related events to the FDA. Besides hospitals, device-user facilities include ambulatory surgical facilities, nursing homes, or outpatient diagnostic or treatment facilities. The FDA reviews all reports it receives and regularly publishes alerts regarding the causes of device-related incidents.[75]

Because of the problems involved in gathering voluntarily reported patient incident data and ensuring the validity and reliability of the information, organizations have begun to create benchmarking databases that provide facts about the common causes of adverse events. This information is gathered in addition to, or instead of, incident prevalence data. Listed below are examples of these initiatives:

- Studies of critical incidents in anesthesia have been carried out in hospitals located as far apart as Hong Kong, Australia, the United Kingdom, North America, and New Zealand.[76] Through an ongoing analysis of the common events and their associated factors, anesthesiologists have learned how to reduce the incidence of similar incidents through improved equipment design and patient management protocols. In the United States, the American Society of Anesthesiologists funds the Closed Claims Project, which is an in-depth investigation of closed anesthesia malpractice claims designed to identify major areas of loss, patterns of injury, and strategies for prevention.[77]
- The Pediatric Perioperative Cardiac Arrest Registry (POCA), sponsored by the American Academy of Pediatrics' Section on Anesthesiology and the Committee on Professional Liability of the American Society of Anesthesiologists, is an investigation of cardiac arrests and deaths of pediatric patients during administration of, or recovery from, anesthesia designed to identify the possible relationship of anesthesia to these incidents.[78]
- The Institute for Safe Medication Practices (ISMP)[79] provides an independent review of medication errors that have been voluntarily submitted to the Medical Errors Reporting Program sponsored

by the United States Pharmacopeia. Although actual medication error reports remain confidential, information about the common factors causing medication errors and how to reduce such errors is distributed to health care facilities by ISMP through its biweekly *Medication Safety Alert* newsletter and various other educational offerings.

- The Joint Commission has been tracking the occurrence of sentinel events in health care facilities since 1996. The findings of these review activities are regularly summarized and shared with the health care community. For example, after reviewing 20 cases related to the death of patients who were being physically restrained, the Joint Commission found similar root causes for these events: (1) incomplete patient assessments; (2) inadequate care planning; (3) lack of patient observation; (4) insufficient staffing or staff training; and (5) equipment-related factors.[80] Several suggestions were offered by the Joint Commission for preventing and reducing restraint deaths in its *Sentinel Event Alert* newsletter.[81]

- The Harvard Medical System formed a Risk Management Incident Collaborative in 1996 for the purpose of developing a comparative database using consistently defined incidents. The database is being used by participating facilities to identify best practices, implement quality-improvement initiatives, continually measure performance, and reduce incidents. Charles Conklin, director of Health Care Quality at Beth Israel Deaconness Medical Center in Boston, is the leader of the project. Kathleen Dwyer, MSN, of the Harvard Risk Management Foundation, provides technical assistance to the risk managers on this project.[82]

- In 1997 the Veterans Health Administration (VHA) reaffirmed its commitment to patient safety by announcing risk management changes that would facilitate facility- and systemwide learning to reduce untoward outcomes related to medical treatment.[83] One component includes the review of all adverse events from a care site-specific and systemwide focus. These reviews identify the root causes of each incident, the changes in design of systems needed to prevent recurrence, and any appropriate personnel actions. All facility reviews of adverse events are sent to the network office and to VHA headquarters, where they are reviewed to identify (1) the adequacy of the facility review and the appropriateness of the actions taken; (2) the frequency with which particular care delivery systems have been problematic so managers know where the best opportunities for improvement exist; (3) system redesigns that should be adopted throughout the network or nationally; (4) needed changes in network and national policies and procedures; and (5) lessons learned that can be shared throughout the VHA on an intranet database. Other health care systems are developing similar incidence and "lessons learned" databases.

These types of mishap databases can provide important learning opportunities for all health care organizations. Solutions to known patient safety problems will no longer have to be reinvented by every facility. By adopting best practices in common work processes instead of only comparing the outputs of those processes, many adverse incidents can be prevented.

CONCLUSION

This chapter describes the use of performance measurement data in reducing errors in high-risk processes along with important points regarding data collection and analysis. This chapter may lack a singular formula for developing performance measures, but it does raise several fundamental questions about how performance can be measured and improved in different types of health care settings. By addressing each of these questions, organizations will eventually discover the most effective error reduction strategy for their environment. Remember, performance measures tend to be evolutionary rather than revolutionary. No one starts with the perfect set of measures; successful organizations evolve their set of measures.

Measuring performance of high-risk processes with the intention of reducing errors is a multifaceted undertaking. It is possible to use any number of performance measures. Currently there is no industrywide consensus on what safety-critical tasks should be regularly evaluated, and there is no national database of adverse events to serve as a prototype. Therefore, individual health care entities are left to select their own risk-related performance measures. An overall organizational plan as to what are the high-risk processes and safety-critical tasks and where measurement efforts should be directed is needed prior to choosing performance measures. Then, with input from risk management and quality improvement departments, the organization's leaders must decide which performance measures will yield the best data.

What is most important is what the organization does with the performance measure data. Performance data can prompt the decision maker to ask for more information (what happened here?), but the performance measure data do not tell the decision-maker why the data are the way they are. Trend information will not make decisions for the leaders nor will the data cause problem areas to vanish. Dedication and commitment are needed from physicians, managers, and staff. Those people intimately involved in the process must have ownership in the choice of measures, the analysis of performance, and any subsequent improvements.

References

1. J. Reason. *Managing the Risks of Organizational Accidents* (Brookfield, VT: Ashgate Publishing Co., 1997), p. 125.

2. P. L. Spath. *Cancer Patient Care Evaluation II: A Fascicle* (Chicago: American College of Surgeons' Commission on Cancer, 1987), p. 24.

3. J. F. Monagle. *Risk Management: A Guide for Health Care Professionals* (Rockville, MD: Aspen Publications, 1985).

4. Physician Insurers Association of America. *Acute Myocardial Infarction Study* (Rockville, MD: PIAA, 1996).

5. Physician Insurers Association of America. *Breast Cancer Study* (Rockville, MD: PIAA, June 1995).

6. Physician Insurers Association of America. *Radiology Practice Standards Claims Survey* (Reston, VA: American College of Radiology, February 1997).

7. Physician Insurers Association of America. *Medication Error Study* (Rockville, MD: PIAA, June 1993).

8. L. B. Andrews et al. "An Alternative Strategy for Studying Adverse Events in Medical Care," *Lancet* 349, no. 9048 (February 1, 1997): 309–13.

9. F. Lefevre et al. "Iatrogenic Complications in High-Risk, Elderly Patients," *Arch Intern Med* 152, no. 10 (October 1992): 2074–80.

10. L. Reed, M. A. Blegen, and C. S. Goode. "Adverse Patient Occurrences as a Measure of Nursing Care Quality," *J Nurs Admin* 28, no. 5 (May 1998): 62–69.

11. J. F. Groves, P. W. Lavori, and J. F. Rosenbaum. "In-Hospital Injuries of Medical and Surgical Patients: The Predictive Effect of a Prior Injury," *Psychosom Med* 54, no. 3 (May-June 1992): 264–74.

12. Total number and type of sentinel events reviewed by the Joint Commission since January 1995. WWW document: http://www.jcaho.org/sentinel?se_stats.htm (January 8, 1999).

13. D. Cave. "Today's Managed Care Market Managing Chronic Disease Patients," *Compensation & Benefits Management* 3, no. 3 (summer 1994): 2–3.

14. T. Giraud et al. "Iatrogenic Complications in Adult Intensive Care Units: A Prospective Two-Center Study," *Crit Care Med* 21, no. 1 (January 1993): 40–51.

15. L. L. Leape et al. "The Nature of Adverse Events in Hospitalized Patients. Results of the Harvard Medical Practice Study II," *N Engl J Med* 324, no. 6 (February 7, 1991): 377–84.

16. T. S. Lesar, B. M. Lomaestro, and H. Pohl. "Medication-Prescribing in a Teaching Hospital: A 9-Year Experience," *Arch Intern Med* 156, no. X (1997): 1569–76.

17. Pharmaceutical Society of Australia. "Current Issues: Pharmacists Welcome Veterans' Medication Program" (September 25, 1977), WWW document: URL: http://www.pas.org.au/issues/25sep97.htm.

18. J. T. Hanlon et al. "Adverse Drug Events in High Risk Older Outpatients," *J Am Geriatr Soc* 45, no. 8 (August 1997): 945–48.

19. Summarized from 1998 issues of the *ISMP Medication Safety Alert* newsletter published by the Institute for Safe Medication Practices, Warminster, PA.

20. A. Kobs. "What's New for 1999? Part III," *Nursing Management* 29, no. 11 (November 1998): 18.

21. Center for Quality of Care Research and Education, Harvard School of Public Health; Mikalix & Company. *CONQUEST 1.0 User's Guide* (Rockville, MD: Agency for Health Care Policy and Research, Department of Health and Human Services, 1996), pp. 3–4.

22. Joint Commission on Accreditation of Healthcare Organizations. *1997–98 Standards for Behavioral Health Care* (Oakbrook Terrace, IL: JCAHO, 1997): 144–45.

23. A. Donabedian. *Explorations in Quality Assessment and Monitoring, Volume I: The Definition of Quality and Approaches to its Assessment* (Ann Arbor, MI: Health Administration Press, 1980).

24. L. B. Andrews et al. "An Alternative Strategy for Studying Adverse Events in Medical Care," pp. 309–13.

25. Food and Drug Administration. "Medical Device Reporting: Manufacturer Reporting, Importer Reporting, User Facility Reporting, and Distributor Reporting," Direct Final Rule, *Federal Register* 63, no. 91 (1998): 26069–77. To be codified at 21 C.F.R. parts 803 and 804.

26. Joint Commission on Accreditation of Healthcare Organizations. "Comprehensive Accreditation Manual for Hospitals, Update 3" (August 1998): PI-6.

27. NASA Lewis Research Center, Office of Safety and Mission. *NASA Guidebook for Safety Critical Software: Analysis and Development* (Washington, DC: National Aeronautics and Space Administration, 1996) (NASA-GB-1740.13-96).

28. B. Wakefield, "Management Culture and Medication Error Reporting," conference presentation, Health Services Research: Implications for Policy, Delivery and Practice, Washington, DC (June 22, 1998).

29. Board of Nurse Examiners for the State of Texas. Rules and Regulations Relating to Professional Nurse Education, Licensure and Practice (October 1998): D25–26.

30. L. L. Leape. "Faulty Systems, Not Faulty People," *The Boston Globe* (January 12, 1999): A15.

31. M. Cohen. "Massachusetts Board Action Will Hurt Patients," *ISMP Medication Safety Alert* 4, no. 1 (January 13, 1998): 1.

32. L. L. Leape et al. "Systems Analysis of Adverse Drug Events," *JAMA* 274, no. X (1995): 35–43.

33. D. Pennachio. "Error Reporting Does a Turn-Around," *Hospital Peer Review* 23, no. 7 (July 1998): 121–23.

34. J. Reason. *Managing the Risks of Organizational Accidents*, p. 197.

35. Institute for Healthcare Improvement. "The Quest for Error-Proof Medicine," *Drug Benefit Trends* 9, no. 6 (1997): 18, 23, 27–29.

36. American Society of Health-System Pharmacists. "Suggested Definitions and Relationships among Medication Misadventures, Medication Errors, Adverse Drug Events, and Adverse Drug Reactions" (September 24, 1997), unpublished document.

37. D. J. Wheeler. *Understanding Variation: The Key to Managing Chaos* (Knoxville, TN: SPC Press, Inc., 1993): 81–105.

38. ECRI. "Risk and Quality Management Strategies: Identifying and Managing Risks," *Healthcare Risk Control* 2 (Plymouth Meeting, PA: ECRI, 1996).

39. D. H. Leeuwen. "Are Medication Error Rates Useful as Comparative Measures of Organizational Performance?" *Journal on Quality Improvement* 20, no. 4 (April 1994): 198.

40. National Coordinating Council for Medication Error Reporting and Prevention (NCC MERP). *Taxonomy of Medication Errors* (NCC MERP of the United States Pharmacopeia, November 1998).

41. H. Baker. "Rules Outside the Rules for Administration of Medications: A Study in New South Wales, Australia," *Journal of Nursing Scholarship* 29, no. 2 (1997): 155–58.

42. G. Fischer et al. "Adverse Events in Primary Care Identified from a Risk-Management Database," *J Fam Pract* 45, no. 1 (July 1997): 40–46.

43. R. L. Kravitz et al. "Malpractice Claims Data as a Quality Improvement Tool, I and II," *JAMA* 266, no. 5 (1991): 2087–97.

44. J. E. Rolph, R. L. Kravitz, and K. McGuigan. "Malpractice Claims Data as a Quality Improvement Tool. II: Is Targeting Effective?" *JAMA* 266, no. 15 (October 1991): 2093–97.

45. D. A. O'Hara and N. J. Carson. "Reporting Adverse Events in Hospitals in Victoria, 1994–1995," *Med J Aust* 166, no. 9 (May 5, 1997): 460–63.

46. C. G. Puckett. *1999 Annual Hospital Version: The Educational Annotation of ICD-9-CM* (Reno, NV: Channel Publishing, Ltd., 1998): 571–76.

47. A. Lawthers, "The Challenge of Identifying In-Hospital Complications from Claims Data," conference presentation, Health Services Research: Implications for Policy, Delivery and Practice, Washington, DC (June 22, 1998).

48. D. W. Bates et al. "Evaluation of Screening Criteria for Adverse Events in Medical Patients," *Medical Care* 33, no. 5 (May 1995): 452–62.

49. Health Care Financing Administration. "Rule for Resident Assessment in Long Term Care Facilities" (42 C.F.R., Part 483), *Federal Register* (December 23, 1997).

50. National Association for Home Care. *Outcome-Based Quality Improvement: A Manual for Home Care Agencies on How to Use Outcomes* (Washington, DC: NAHC, 1995).

51. L. A. Norman and P. A. Hardin. "Computer-Assisted Outcomes Management in the Ambulatory Care Setting," in P. Spath, ed., *Medical Effectiveness and Outcomes Management: Issues, Methods, and Case Studies* (Chicago: American Hospital Publishing, Inc., 1996), pp. 313–16.

52. D. W. Bates et al. "Evaluation of Screening Criteria for Adverse Events in Medical Patients," pp. 452–62.

53. C. Klassen, ART, Quality Improvement Coordinator and Information Management Director, University Neuropsychiatric Institute, interview with author (P. Spath), Salt Lake City, UT (July 1998).

54. T. A. Brennan, R. J. Localio, and N. L. Laird. "Reliability and Validity of Judgments Concerning Adverse Events Suffered by Hospitalized Patients," *Medical Care* 27, no. 12 (December 1989): 1148–58.

55. P. L. Spath. "Plan for Data Collection," *Hospital Peer Review* 23, no. 11 (November 1998): 207–10.

56. D. A. Tribble et al. "Ideas for Action: Reporting Medication Error Rate by Microcomputer," *Topics in Hospital Pharmacy Management* 5, no. 1 (1985): 77–88.

57. D. H. Leeuwen. "Are Medication Error Rates Useful as Comparative Measures of Organizational Performance?" pp. 192–99.

58. J. C. Bauer. *Statistical Analysis for Decision Makers in Healthcare* (Chicago: Irwin Professional Publishing, 1996), pp. 39–56.

59. O. R. Ellis and C. E. Schfiling. *Process Quality Control, Troubleshooting and Interpretation of Data* (New York: MGraw-Hill, 1990), pp. 44–56.

60. D. J. Wheeler and D. S. Chambers. *Understanding Statistical Process Control*, 2d ed. (Knoxville, TN: SPC Press, 1992).

61. M. Pelling and M. Smith. "Data-Driven Outcomes Management," in P. Spath, ed., *Medical Effectiveness and Outcomes Management: Issues, Methods, and Case Studies*, pp. 20–21.

62. Executive Learning Inc. *Continual Improvement Handbook: A Quick Reference Guide for Tools and Concepts, Healthcare Version* (Brentwood, TN: Executive Learning, Inc., 1993), pp. 6–17.

63. R. G. Gift and D. Mosel. *Benchmarking in Health Care* (Chicago: American Hospital Publishing, Inc., 1994), p. 5.

64. R. H. Ogle. "Benchmarking: A Path to Excellence," conference presentation, Benchmarking: The Next Generation in Healthcare Quality, Chicago (September 18, 1992).

65. Center for Quality of Care Research and Education, Harvard School of Public Health Final Report: CONQUEST 1.0. *A COmputerized Needs-oriented QUality measurement Evaluation SysTem* (Rockville, MD: Department of Health and Human Services, Public Health Service, Agency for Health Care Policy and Research, 1996), p. 4.

66. D. W. Bates, L. Leape, and S. Petrycki. "Drug-Related Adverse Events in Hospitalized Patients," *Clin Research* 39, no. 4 (1991): 596A.

67. E. L. Allan and K. N. Barker. "Fundamentals of Medication Error Research," *American Journal of Hospital Pharmacy* 47, no. 3 (1990): 555–71.

68. L. B. Andrews et al. "An Alternative Strategy for Studying Adverse Events in Medical Care," pp. 309–13.

69. J. B. Fitzmaurice. "Reducing Risks for Falls," *Newsletter of the Harvard Risk Management Foundation* (March 1993).

70. J. M. Geiduschek. "Registry Offers Insight on Preventing Cardiac Arrests in Children," *ASA Newsletter* 62, no. 6 (1998): 16–18.

71. M. R. Yessian. "Putting the Controversy Aside, How Is the Data Bank Doing?" *Public Health Reports* (July 1995).

72. M. Green and G. von Nostitz. *What the State Health Department Doesn't Know Could Hurt You: How NYC Hospitals Fail to Report Poor Care* (New York: The Public Advocate's Office, April 1998).

73. Ibid., p. 42.

74. C. Billings. "Incident Reporting Systems in Medicine and Experience with the Aviation Safety Reporting System," conference presentation, Assembling the Scientific Basis for Progress on Patient Safety, Chicago (December 16, 1997).

75. The complete files of reports received under the Medical Devices Reporting Program from 1984–1996 are available on the Web at: http://www.fda.gov/cdrh/mdrfile.html. More recent reports can be found at http://www.fda.gov/cdrh/.

76. M. C. Derrington. "Critical Incidents in Anaesthesia," in J. S. Walker, ed., *Quality and Safety in Anaesthesia* (London: BMJ Publishing Group, 1994), p. 113.

77. For more information about the patient safety activities of the American Society of Anesthesiologists, visit its Web site at: http://apsf.med.yale.edu/.

78. For more information about the Pediatric Perioperative Cardiac Arrest Registry, visit its Web site at: http://weber.u.washington.edu/~asaccp/.

79. For more information about the Institute for Safe Medication Practices, visit its Web site at: http://www.ismp.org.

80. Joint Commission on Accreditation of Healthcare Organizations. *Sentinel Event Alert* 9 (November 18, 1998), WWW document: http://www.jcaho.org/pubedmul/publicat/sealert/se_alert.htm (printed January 16, 1999).

81. For more information on the Joint Commission's *Sentinel Event Alert* newsletter, visit its Web site at: http://www.jcaho.org.

82. Risk Management Foundation. *Resource*, monthly audiotape (April 1998).

83. Department of Veterans Affairs. *Veterans Health Administration Patient Safety Handbook*, VHA Directive 1051/1 (Washington, DC: Department of Veterans Affairs, 1998).

3

The Human Side of Medical Mistakes

Sven Ternov, MD

hether it be an automobile assembly plant or a hospital, a production system consists of a lot of organized activities whose aim is to add value to whatever is put into the system. A production system is made up of human operators who use different kinds of equipment and who cooperate in a structured way. The different activities in the system are often called *processes*. The processes take place inside an *organization*. The organization contains the framework of rules for how groups of human operators and equipment shall cooperate to achieve the production goals of the organization. When these interdependent activities reach a certain volume, the system can be labeled a *complex system*.

Over the past decade researchers have made tremendous advances toward understanding and correcting the causes of accident behavior in complex technical systems (for example, nuclear power, air and rail traffic, and shipping). Similar advances in the health care industry have been slow to materialize. Perhaps this is because medical accidents do not get the same headlines and public attention as the megadisaster. Health care accidents cause one death at a time, not the several hundred that might result from a major airline crash.

Current concepts in modern risk management suggest that accidents in complex systems basically result from interface problems (*human-system misfits*). In air traffic control, for example, 80 to 90 percent of accidents have been found to be caused by human malfunctions rather than technical causes.[1] Figures for the medical domain point in the same direction; with Chopra and others having found human malfunction as the cause for adverse patient outcomes in 70 percent of cases[2] and Cooper and others reporting human-related causes in 82 percent of medical accidents.[3]

To prevent the unexpected and undesirable patient outcomes that may result from these human-system misfits, health care providers must have a better understanding of humans as problem solvers in a complex system, the interface between humans and the systems in which they function, and how humans exert influence on the system. In the first part of this chapter, readers will learn more about how people make decisions and why social and system influences can cause human errors.

The term *error* itself can be criticized as being imprecise and a hindsight judgment. We do not know what becomes an error before we see the effect of the faulty action. If the system safeguards can absorb the effect of a faulty human action or if we have good luck, then there is no error. With poor system defenses or sheer bad luck, the same faulty action is labeled an error. Whether or not a clumsy human action is ultimately determined to be an error is primarily beyond the human's control. This determination is primarily affected by the design of the system in which the human is working and sheer fate. Throughout this chapter actual case studies from the files of the Swedish National Board of Health and Welfare are used to illustrate how ineffectual system safeguards and other human-system misfits magnify the consequences of faulty human actions.

What is known about the human-system interface can be applied to the retrospective analysis of medical mistakes. In the context of this chapter, a medical mistake is considered to be a faulty human action made during the diagnosis or treatment of a patient that results in damage to, or death of, the patient. Other terms often used to describe these incidents are *untoward event, sentinel event,* and *accident.* In the latter half of the chapter, readers will be introduced to MTO Analysis (the abbreviation MTO stands for Man-Technique-Organization). This is an accident investigation method originally developed by NASA and later adopted by the American nuclear power industry. It has been adopted by the Swedish nuclear power industry and has been adapted for use by the Swedish National Board of Health and Welfare to examine medical mistakes. MTO analysis helps investigators identify the human-system problems that contributed to the accident, find the underlying causes of the accident, and develop preventive actions. Swedish researchers such as myself have also begun to apply the principles of

MTO Analysis in a proactive manner to identify and resolve medical process problems before an undesirable patient outcome occurs. Although this work is in its preliminary stages, a brief explanation of such an analysis will be presented.

HUMANS AS PROBLEM SOLVERS

Certain elements in cognitive psychology are essential building blocks in understanding how humans solve problems and why mistakes occur. These elements are the concepts of *long-term memory* and *working memory, chunking* (of information), the *schemata model* for storage and retrieval of knowledge, and models concerning limitation of *attention*. These cognitive elements have varying influences on human performance at different levels of problem solving. As the amount of cognitive processing resources needed by a human to solve a problem increases, the greater the likelihood of a mistake. The environment also influences the reliability of problem solving. Less-than-desirable work situations and stressful personal circumstances can greatly increase the chance of a mistake. In this section, readers are introduced to the cognitive and environmental factors that influence how humans solve problems.

Long-Term and Working Memory

Long-term memory is a sort of knowledge database with seemingly unlimited capacity. This is contrary to the former (and popular) notion that "the brain" has a limited capacity to store knowledge (if something went in, something else had to be thrown out). As readers of the Sherlock Holmes stories by Sir Arthur Conan Doyle may remember, the famous crime investigator used this notion as an excuse for not bothering with learning trivia like the prices of groceries, how to cook, and the like. He wanted to use his limited and valuable "brain space" to store knowledge on how to distinguish between 50 different types of cigar ashes and a lot of other peculiar knowledge necessary for his deductional powers. He was wrong. The long-term memory works quickly and without cognitive effort. It can process parallel bits of information and knowledge retrieval is mainly subconscious.

Working memory, on the contrary, is slow and conscious. Working memory can only process one thing at a time and has a very limited capacity. The working memory is necessary for directing our attention to that part of a problem we are consciously dealing with. If we try to direct our attention to too many problems at a time, the working memory gets overloaded. To prevent this from occurring, humans tend to focus their attention. Unfortunately, this can lead to attentional "lock-up" on the wrong part of the problem. The following three case studies illustrate what can happen when a medical professional is reluctant to switch attention once he or she has zoomed in on what is perceived to be the problem.[4]

Case Study #1: Missed diagnosis of pheochromocytoma
A doctor (a very distinguished professor and specialist on pheochromocytoma) got a referral from a general practitioner (GP) concerning a 40-year-old man. The patient had a high blood pressure that was very labile and difficult to treat. He also had a very interesting and dramatic psychosocial background, which easily might have explained his oscillating blood pressure and even other symptoms such as attacks of dizziness and flushing. All the signs were interpreted by the specialist as favoring the psychosomatic explanation. After several months the patient happened to see his GP again. She ordered a laboratory test of adrenaline metabolites in the blood and in a few days she had made the correct diagnosis of pheochromocytoma. The patient was successfully treated and the professor was highly embarrassed.

Case Study #2: Missed diagnosis of nephrotic syndrome
An older patient was treated at a department of internal medicine for edema of the lower legs. The swelling was very resistant to treatment with diuretics. Furthermore, the patient's kidneys showed signs of not functioning very well, so the doctor very carefully followed the patient's creatinine levels on the computer printout of laboratory test results. Had the doctor just raised his gaze one inch on the test report he might have noticed a row of five consecutive blood analyses showing a very low serum albumin caused, of course, by the patient's nephrotic syndrome.

Case Study #3: Missed diagnosis of diabetic ketoacidosis
An elderly gentleman was brought to the emergency department complaining of breathing difficulties. He had a known asthmatic

condition; however, the medication he took at home had not brought relief to his symptoms. On physical examination the expected findings of wheezing were heard on the lungs, which disappeared with the usual infusion of asthma drugs. The patient's breathing difficulties, however, got only slightly better. The patient was admitted to an inpatient bed. X-ray studies of the patient's lungs did not show anything special and his condition remained a puzzle to several physicians.

After some hours a new doctor came on duty. Upon entering the patient's room, she immediately smelled acetone and located the laboratory test in the patient's chart, which revealed the patient's high blood glucose level and a very pathological acid-base balance. Within 30 seconds this physician made the correct diagnosis of diabetic ketoacidosis. The physicians who had earlier treated the patient had their attention on the wrong condition. The asthma "label" followed the patient for hours before the real diagnosis was discovered.

Chunking of Information

According to one of several models in cognitive psychology, knowledge is stored in the long-term memory in chunks of information called *schematas* (or scripts or frames). Schematas contain knowledge structured in a functional way so that it is retrieved in a ready-to-use fashion and is made up of one's previous experience of similar situations. The schematas are stored in a hierarchical system with main rules for solving a problem (for instance a diagnostic problem) on the top, with siderules and exceptions from the rules further down in the hierarchy. The novice has only a limited number of schematas with main rules, but the expert problem solver has stored a lot of side rules and exceptions from the main rules.

Schematas have different strengths. A strong schema is more readily retrieved (and applied) than a weak one. What makes a schema strong is how recently and how frequently it has been used. That is, if a problem solver often uses solution A to a problem, the chances are high that he or she will use solution A instead of solution B even if solution B is the better choice or solution A downright wrong. The case study below illustrates how a physician's strong schema was unfortunately not the right choice.

Case Study #4: The wrong method for anesthesia is used and the patient dies.

A 42-year-old women underwent a partial thyroidectomy. Shortly after the operation she shows signs of developing a hematoma in the wound area. The surgeon and the patient's nurse monitor this situation carefully for the next four hours. The surgeon finally decides to bring the patient back to the operating room for removal of the hematoma. He notifies the anesthesiologist by phone and later has a very short oral communication with him in a corridor outside the operating room. The surgeon then goes off to attend to some other matter and leaves the anesthesiologist in charge of the patient. The patient is doing fairly well and can talk to the anesthesiologist.

The anesthesiologist believes it best to intubate the patient right away. He starts an IV line, administers muscle relaxant, and then attempts to intubate the patient. The intubation is not successful and he tries to ventilate the patient with a mask, which also fails. He makes a new attempt to intubate the patient and initially believes the tube is in the patient's trachea, but after another minute finds the second intubation is also a failure. Now the surgeon has arrived and a lot of other staff as well. Some debate is going on between surgeon and anesthesiologist whether or not the patient is properly intubated. The situation is close to panic. After six minutes and more attempts, successful ventilation is finally established, but this is too late and the patient expires.

Comments: The anesthesiologist performed the intubation the way he was used to doing it; that is, he gave the patient a muscle relaxant and then intubated. He used a rule that he very frequently used to solve this kind of problem and thus the rule was strong. But it was also a wrong rule. In anesthesiology it is well known that intubation of patients with neck and throat disorders is very tricky and dangerous because of the swelling in the throat. Relaxing the muscles in the throat with muscle relaxant makes it even more difficult to intubate, and in case of intubation failure these patients can be very difficult to ventilate on a mask. Since their spontaneous breathing is paralyzed by the muscle relaxant, the danger is very great that they get anoxic.

Instead, he should have used induction with gas or, better yet, had an ENT specialist stand by for intubation with fiberscope. The anesthesiologist had a poor understanding of the situation, causing him to "read" the wrong cues. It might have helped if the surgeon had better conveyed to the anesthesiologist the patient's background and the dynamics of the problem. Because of lack of communication, the problem got cognitively underspecified (see below) for the anesthesiologist—a common cause for reading a problem wrong.

The use of a "strong-but-wrong" schema is not the whole explanation for the tragic outcome described above. Many things must, as a rule, go wrong before a patient is lost. This was also the case in this accident. Among other problems, the equipment for monitoring carbon dioxide in the patient's expiratory air was missing, thus delaying the detection of esophageal intubation.

A schema is also (subconsciously) chosen if it is similar to the current problem situation. This similarity matching[5] creates another great possibility for error because the problem solver might read the problem situation wrong; that is, the features toward which he or she directs attention might be the wrong cues to the problem. Thus, the similarity matching tries to retrieve a rule that matches these (wrong) cues. Subsequently, the retrieved rule is wrong for solving the actual problem. Given sufficient time and working memory capacity, the problem solver may detect this; otherwise, the risk is great that a faulty action will occur (as in case study #4).

To misread a problem is a common cause of error. Often we direct our attention to more salient features that are not necessarily the same as the important features. In case study #3 the salient feature was the asthmatic condition and in case study #1 it was the patient's dramatic psychosocial background. When we direct our limited attentional resources to the wrong cues, the problem might be said to be *cognitive underspecified*[6] (as in case study #4). A problem can get underspecified for several reasons—common factors are time pressures and attempting to focus our attention on too many problems at once. It is also more difficult for a novice to identify the proper cues in a problem situation compared with an expert.

Sometimes errors occur because the problem is ill defined rather than cognitively underspecified. To perform well, the person should know the start-state and end-state of a problem. However, the start-state of real-life problems are often ill defined, causing us to miss the real problem. This situation is illustrated in case study #5 below.

**Case Study #5: Destruction of the seventh cervical vertebra
is not noticed by the radiologist.**
A radiologist gets a referral from a GP for x-ray examination of the
cervical column on a patient who presents with the common complaint of neck and shoulder pain. The GP writes "spondylosis?" on
the referral slip. It only takes half a minute for the radiologist to find
x-ray evidence for this diagnosis; thus, the answer to the GP's asked
question is "yes!" Fourteen days later the patient comes to the emergency department because of worsening pain. This time an MRI is
done. It shows destruction of more than half of the seventh cervical
vertebra. On reexamination of the original x-ray, this destruction is
clearly evident.

Did the radiologist commit an error when interpreting the first x-
ray? This question can be answered in different ways. One could say
that the problem was underspecified for the radiologist at the first
examination. He used rule-based problem solving and retrieved a
schema from his long-term memory that was labeled: "Do these pictures
show spondylosis, yes or no?" One might argue that he instead should
have used a different schema: "Is this cervical column healthy or not?"
But the start-state of the problem was not defined for him in this way,
making the problem ill defined from the very beginning.

Once we know the end-state—knowledge about destruction of a
vertebra (which turned out to be a metastasis from a kidney tumor)—
we can, in hindsight, define the start-state properly. It should have been:
"Are there any signs of destruction of the vertical column that might
explain the symptoms?" Because the radiologist did not have this hindsight information when interpreting the original x-ray, his initial reading
should not be categorized as an error. In my opinion the problem was ill
defined for the radiologist.

James Reason mentions another error mechanism, *confirmation
bias*, that partly contributes to medical mistakes.[7] Confirmation bias
works like this. When we have decided on a course of action (we have
retrieved a schema with a strong rule), we stick firmly to this choice.
New information that really is contradictory to the chosen course of
action is (subconsciously) disregarded or, where possible, interpreted
in favor of our choice. Woods uses the term *cognitive fixation* to
describe these phenomena.[8] A synonymous term is *cognitive lock-up*.
Confirmation bias appears to be a common reason for medical mistakes, as illustrated by case study #6 below.

Case Study #6: Missed diagnosis of a perforated ulcer

A 22-year-old male patient who is slightly mentally retarded is brought to the emergency department by his mother following the rapid onset of abdominal pain. The mother, who is very informative, quickly volunteers the information that about a year ago her son had a ureteric stone condition and that his current complaints are very much the same. Physical examination and laboratory tests of blood and urine do not show anything conclusive.

The doctor treats the patient for urinary stones. The patient receives an injection of analgesics, is observed for a few hours, and then receives another injection. After three hours the patient improves and is taken home by his mother. The next morning the patient suddenly dies. Autopsy reveals a perforated duodenal ulcer.

Comments: Strongly influenced by the patient's history provided by his mother, in a matter of minutes the physician made up his mind about what was wrong with the patient. New information (laboratory tests, patient's response to treatment) is interpreted by the doctor as favoring the ureteric stone diagnosis. The absence of hematuria does not necessarily contradict this diagnosis and the physician finds that the patient reacts to treatment in the usual way.

In the harsh light of hindsight, the physician should have counteracted the threat of confirmation bias using reasoning such as, "Absence of hematuria doesn't contradict my diagnosis, but it doesn't support it either. Could the patient have some other condition? The patient reacts to the analgesics the way I expect him to, but this same response would be expected for other abdominal conditions that I might have overlooked. Which conditions must I think of, and exclude, before I allow him to return home?"

Skill-, Rule-, and Knowledge-Based Problem Solving

After studying the operators who control complex technical systems (mainly nuclear power), Rasmussen and other authors have suggested that human problem solving can be categorized into the following three levels:[9]

1. Skill based
2. Rule based
3. Knowledge based

Skill-based problem solving is used with highly automated work processes, based on stereotypical motor movements like working at an assembly line. *Rule-based* problem solving is used in novel situations, in which we recognize features from similar situations. Here we use ready-made solutions retrieved from long-term memory. We use *knowledge-based* problem solving in novel situations in which we are not able to identify features that resemble something we have done before; that is, we are not able to retrieve a rule/schema with a ready solution to the problem. In knowledge-based problem solving it appears that we try to restructure the problem to give us hints as to which ready-made solutions from our long-term memory could be applied in this situation.

Errors can occur in each of these problem-solving levels. Errors in skill-based problem solving emanate from the automatic nature of motor movements. The work is mainly done without conscious control, like driving a car along a highway under favorable conditions. At certain times it is necessary to apply conscious control to ensure that the automatic actions proceed as intended; for example, you pay closer attention when you reach the desired highway exit. If this control node is missed, you will find yourself speeding past the exit. These conscious control nodes are very sensitive to distraction (like a talkative passenger in the car). A health care example of a skill-based problem-solving error is illustrated in case study #7 below.

Case Study #7: Midwife takes the wrong drug vial off the shelf.
A midwife intends to give a pregnant woman with premature labor an infusion of a drug that inhibits labor. At the moment when she is going to take the vial from the shelf, she is distracted by a question from a colleague. She continues her intended action but chooses instead a vial containing a drug that stimulates labor. Fortunately, she discovers her mistake when she does the last procedural check before coupling the infusion set to the patient's intravenous line.

Comments: The same motor schema is used by the midwife whether she is taking vial A or vial B from the same storage shelf. In this case the control node is missing because of the midwife's distraction. Thankfully, the mistake was caught before a harmful incident occurred.

Examples of error mechanisms in rule-based problem solving have been discussed earlier in this section (how one uses the wrong rules and confirmation bias). However, there is another mechanism in rule-based problem solving that needs to be presented. Rasmussen suggests that the human operator's fantastic ability to *adapt* to various situations can be a source of errors.[10] The human's ability to adapt to the peculiarities of various systems makes us very efficient controllers of systems; however, this ability makes us much more vulnerable to errors. Trade-offs that may be necessary when working within a system can cause us to adopt less safe ways of doing things (cutting corners). A health care example of this mechanism at work is illustrated in case study #8.

Case Study #8: Caregiver adopts the wrong rule.

During a patient's preoperative assessment, the anesthesiologist discovers that the patient has a condition that might endanger her safety during anesthesia. The anesthesiologist believes the condition should be investigated further before surgery is undertaken. However, the investigation will delay the planned procedure, and the anesthesiologist knows he will be intimidated by the surgeon for such a recommendation ("Be a man, don't fuss, let's get on with it," or if a female anesthesiologist, "Typical woman!"). So the anesthesiologist finds himself in a trade-off situation. Should he play it safe or keep the surgeon happy? The anesthesiologist decides to take the easy way out and does not proceed with further investigations of the patient's condition. The surgery commences as originally planned and luckily the patient does not experience an anesthetic mishap.

The next time the anesthesiologist encounters a similar situation, the easy way might again be chosen, this time with less deliberation. After a while the anesthesiologist might have adopted a strong, but not so good, rule. Some day this rule could prove to be strong but wrong if the patient suffers an adverse outcome.

Error mechanisms in knowledge-based problem solving occur when the human's working memory has to bear the whole burden of problem solving. With the limited capacity of the working memory, the probability increases that one's attention will be directed to a less important part of the problem. Likewise, important parts of the problem might be missed because knowledge-based problem solving is time consuming, and time is very limited in dynamic medical situations. Case #10 (ahead on page 116) gives a good illustration of this error mechanism. In this instance a night nurse in a geriatric long-term care unit is ordered to prepare an elderly patient with diabetes for hip surgery the following morning. She has very little experience with pre-operative procedures. Thus her similarity matching for ready-made solutions to the problem gives a meager result. She has to rely on her limited working memory resources, slowly, serially, and meticulously working her way through the problem. During the hours of early morning when she finally is expected to prepare an insulin infusion, her working memory resources are depleted and she administers 10 times the prescribed amount of insulin to the patient.

System Factors Influencing Problem Solving

While the cognitive aspects of problem solving have a significant impact, these aspects do not by themselves explain why medical mistakes occur. External factors—so-called *performance shaping factors*—can have great negative impact on our problem-solving ability. Typical factors are stress, time pressure, distraction, goal conflicts, and physical factors (like temperature and noise). Internal factors, such as one's personal problems and level of training, will also influence how we perform.

The majority of these performance-shaping factors are heavily influenced by management decisions and, as such, are generally beyond the control of the individual operator.

Apart from internal and external performance-shaping factors, the way a problem is presented to the operator can be a negative system factor. To eliminate these negative system factors, the *problem space* should be redesigned in such a manner as to reduce the operator's cognitive workload. For example, the problem-solving processes that occur during complicated treatment regimens (such as administration of cytotoxic agents) can place a heavy cognitive burden on clinicians. Computer technology that calculates drug dosages and keeps track of the time for the next treatment, next blood sample, and so on can lessen the cognitive workload of the operators.

THE HUMAN-SYSTEM INTERFACE

Just like a nuclear power plant, a hospital or a department within the hospital can be considered a system. In the power plant, the system is made up of staff, core, turbines, and buildings. A health care system consists of staff, equipment, buildings, and the patient who is receiving treatment.

A system can be more or less stable. A stable system performs the way it is supposed to; for example, the production runs smoothly and produces electrical power or treated patients without mishaps every time and all the time. The processes in a stable system are considered to be *reliable* and *safe*. Various factors can cause the system state to become unstable, thus causing the processes to become *unreliable* and *unsafe*. The system can move into a state of *lack of control*, which can proceed to a *loss-of-control state* if no corrective actions are taken; *system failure* is imminent. A health care system failure can lead to serious injury or death of a patient.

The health care production system has many similarities to other complex systems, but substantial differences also exist. Thus, knowledge gleaned from studies of the behavior of complex technical systems should be applied cautiously to health care. Listed below are the considerations that must be taken into account when technical systems theory is applied to the health care environment.

- Compared to technical systems, health care is a much more personnel-intensive and personnel-driven system. Authors have called health care a sociotechnical system.[11] In nuclear power and aviation, for instance, the people are largely supervisors of automated processes. The health care system is largely composed of processes conducted by the people themselves.
- The health care system is made up of numerous autonomous units or disciplines, each having its own rules, procedures, and cultures. The people in each discipline must cooperate in achieving the same goal (treatment of a patient). Informal oral communication within and between these units plays a major role in health care processes, whereas many technical systems rely heavily on large volumes of written instructions to guide processes.

- In health care, information about system changes are communicated horizontally among caregivers, often with little structure for how changes shall take place. Changes in a technical system are often mediated vertically in a strict hierarchical organization. Thus, changes in health care processes will often be slow and unreliable, thereby endangering system safety. With this reflection I do not mean to claim that the technical way is the best on all occasions. It has its drawbacks, too; for instance, operators get fed up with an endless flow of written procedures, with the final instruction being one that stresses the importance of reading all the other instructions!
- In health care, the relationship between an action and the effect of the action is often less precise than for technical systems. If, for instance, an operator in a nuclear power plant wrongly closes a valve that depletes the core of its coolant, the effect is very certain—the core temperature will rise. If a radiologist gives the wrong diagnostic conclusion following an x-ray examination (like the event mentioned in case study #5 on page 104), the effect is less certain. It might create a system failure. However, the recipient of the radiologist's report might question the answer, or the answer may not significantly influence future patient treatment decisions. Thus the health care system is called *loosely coupled*, while technical systems often are *tightly coupled*. This loose relationship between an action and the effect of the action makes health care risk management more of a qualitative than a quantitative exercise.

System Behavior in Accidents

Following the investigations of several past disasters (such as the Challenger shuttle explosion, the nuclear accidents at Three Mile Island and Chernobyl, the Bhopal chemical plant disaster, King's Cross metro station fire, and the Exxon Valdez oil spill in Alaska), a research model has surfaced to explain why errors occur in complex technical systems.[12] Although the health care system might be viewed as slightly different from technical systems, this model has application to the medical environment.

According to this model, errors in a complex system can be divided into two classes: *active failures* and *latent failures*. Errors made by the operators performing the processes fall into the category of active failures. For example, faulty actions by the doctor, the nurse, or any other direct caregiver are considered active failures. In case study #7 (page 106), the midwife taking the wrong medication vial from the storage shelf would be classed as an active failure. Latent failures are attributed to the people who influence the system but who are not active participants; for example, housekeeping, maintenance, information systems, and management. These people are typically very faceless in an accident situation compared with the operators in the system. A latent failure, for example, might be an inappropriately designed medication preparation procedure that creates a potential for pharmacist error.

Many people view the term *root cause* to be synonymous with latent failure. *Root cause* can be a fairly imprecise term when used in a general way to describe causes for erroneous actions that may occur at any point along a chain of events. An example of the various causes that might be identified as the investigator digs deeper into a medical mistake are illustrated in figure 3-1. The types of causes identified in the answers to the first four questions might often be labeled root causes; however, it is not until question 5 that a real root cause or latent system failure is identified. Thus it is a matter of definitions. In my opinion, a cause should not be labeled a root cause (or latent failure) if it does not actually say something about the organization's underlying system for managing the processes (quality system).

Whether *latent failure* or *root cause* is used to describe faults in the underlying systems (such as quality control, communication, information sharing, staff training, allocation of resources, and so on) the description depends on the quality system chosen for referencing the analysis. Personally I prefer the demands from the ISO 9000 international standard for quality management (the ISO 9001 standard for quality assurance).

Often latent failures exist for many years in a system without causing a medical accident. It is usually so-called *situational factors* (also known as *unlucky circumstances*) that activate the latent failures and cause them to exert negative system influences. For example, when the midwife in case study #7 was distracted by a colleague, a latent failure was activated. The procedure that allowed a drug that inhibits labor to be stored on the shelf close to a drug that stimulates labor had never before resulted in a medication error. When the situational factor of distraction was introduced into the system, the latent failure (drug vial

Figure 3-1. Typical Questions Asked during a Medical Accident Investigation

---

Event: A physician makes an error.

Question #1: Why did the physician make an error?

Answer: Because he did not pay sufficient attention to the important part of the problem.

Question #2: Why didn't he pay sufficient attention?

Answer: Because he was stressed (his working memory resources were depleted).

Question #3: Why was he stressed?

Answer: Because he was caring for two acutely ill patients at the same time and he was rather inexperienced.

Question #4: Why did he have to do that? Couldn't he contact someone for help? Was he too inexperienced to be assigned to this work task?

Answer: Well, the senior staff physicians do not like to be disturbed at night. And yes, he was maybe too inexperienced for this kind of patient care assignment.

Question #5: Do you have any procedures regulating the necessary level of training and experience that physicians must have before they are assigned to a particular patient care task?

Answer: No, not really.

---

storage procedure) contributed to the midwife's selecting the wrong drug from the shelf. Another latent failure might be working procedures that do not allow the nurse to prepare medications without interruption.

Once activated, latent failures can trap the operator into committing an active failure, impede error detection, or create messy situations (such as stresses or time pressures) that negatively influence the operator's performance. Even when latent failures are activated, most health care systems have safeguards to prevent errors from causing patient harm. A safety barrier is an administrative or technical constraint that can act in one of two ways. The safety barrier can hinder the operator from committing an active failure or it can absorb the effect of the active failure before it exerts negative system influence. An example of a technical barrier is the manner in which ECG-electrodes are designed to prevent them from being plugged into the main power supply. The physician computer order entry system that requires dosage, route, and frequency be entered for all medication orders is another example of a technical barrier.[13]

A procedure that requires double-checks of information before action is taken (the safeguard in case study #7 that prevented a medication error) is an example of an administrative barrier. Another administrative barrier would be the requirements that the Mayo table set-ups in the operating room are standardized for all procedures.

Safety barriers can be weak or strong and might even be called absolute or relative, depending on the barrier's ability to absorb the effect of, or prevent, active failures. It is easier to make technical barriers absolute, whereas active failures may slip through the cracks of administrative barriers. However, it should be noted that the absoluteness of any safety barrier can be debated with reference to one of Murphy's laws: "You can't make anything foolproof because fools are so ingenious."

The Accident Trajectory

The relationship between situational factors, latent and active failures, and safety barriers in a medical accident is illustrated by the typical accident trajectory in figure 3-2. A real accident situation is far more complex than suggested by this model. It is common to find that several latent failures were activated and these failures interacted with each other in a complicated manner before the system defenses (barriers) were breached to such an extent that a system failure occurred.

Figure 3-2. Typical Medical Accident Trajectory

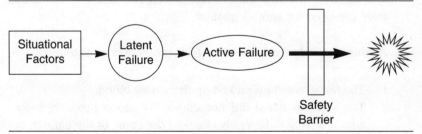

Accidents in complex systems commonly exhibit certain patterns or behaviors that can be summarized like this:

- One or, more frequently, several latent failures are the causes of the accident.
- Latent failures act as error traps, create a messy problem-solving environment, or impede error detection.
- Flaws in the system safety barriers can almost always be demonstrated.
- Situational factors play an important role by triggering the dormant latent failures into activity.

Although the evidence for this model is derived mainly from accident investigations in complex technical systems, there is no reason why it cannot be applied to health care. The following case studies clearly demonstrate these accident behavior characteristics.

Case Study #9: One patient gets another patient's blood.

The setting is an operating room. A patient is undergoing minor elective gynecological surgery under general anesthesia. She suddenly starts to bleed and her blood pressure falls. The patient is given intravenous fluids and blood is ordered from the blood bank. At the same time the patient has an asthma attack that has to be remedied.

A nurse assistant goes to the blood bank, picks up the blood, and delivers it to the operating room. The surgical nurse double-checks the name of the patient against the name on the blood and then transfuses the blood. The patient is stabilized and the operation is completed. After one hour the staff in the postoperative care unit discover that the patient has gotten two units of blood that were intended for another patient.

Accident Analysis: Two *active failures* were committed:

1. The nurse assistant picked up the wrong blood.
2. The surgical nurse did not check the blood properly before administering it. She only checked the name of the patient, not the medical record number as required by procedures.

A *latent failure* leading to the first active failure was a flawed procedure for picking up blood. Only the name of the patient was communicated by the surgical nurse to the nurse assistant. The nurse assistant was not told the patient's medical record number.

Other latent failures contributing to the first active failure involved the procedures used by the blood bank for separating stat blood orders from nonemergent orders and procedures for setting aside blood that has been readied for use but not transfused as intended.

The *situational factor* necessary for this accident evolution was that at this time two patients with the same name were admitted to the same facility at the same time, and the same amount of blood had been ordered for each patient (two units). The blood requested for stat intraoperative use had yet to be placed in the blood bank's refrigerator at the time the nurse assistant arrived in the blood bank (the physician thought the blood would not be needed until after surgery, if at all). However, the nurse assistant saw two units in the refrigerator with the correct patient name and assumed that these were the correct units.

The flawed procedure of not giving the nurse assistant the patient's medical record number to check against the product in the blood bank's refrigerator could also be designated a latent failure. It could, however, be labeled a *flawed safety barrier.* If the nurse assistant were expected to check the patient's medical record number as well as the patient's name, she would probably not have picked up the wrong blood units from the refrigerator. As this situation illustrates, the distinction between a latent failure and a flawed safety barrier can be difficult. The important thing is not the label but that the problem is identified and remedied.

A *latent failure* leading to the second active failure (omitted control before administering the blood) was discovered by examining the problem-solving environment of the surgical nurse. It was found that the system of care in the operating room expected the surgical nurse to regularly function with heavy mental workloads. Although this latent failure may have existed for many years without contributing to a medical accident, an overwhelming number of *situational factors* activated the latent failure and caused it to exert negative system influences.

At the time when the surgical nurse was transfusing the blood, she had a lot of activities going on that placed a heavy burden on the limited resources of her working memory (which controls attention). For example:

- She was worried about the patient's blood pressure and was monitoring it carefully.
- She was carrying out the anesthesiologist's orders concerning treatment of the patient's asthmatic condition.
- At the same time an anesthesiologist from another operating room came into the room and distracted her with questions.
- She was also acting as tutor for a medical student (among other things, teaching her how to check blood before administering it to patients).
- Finally, she was acting as switchboard for this section of the surgical department. She was carrying around a cellular phone in her pocket and the phone was ringing all the time.

Because of these situational factors, the surgical nurse was depleting the limited resources of her working memory. It is easily understood from the description of the circumstances surrounding this event that the nurse did not have much working memory left over to allow her to pay close attention to the procedure of checking the blood. The work task design of having to answer phone calls in such a dynamic environment was deemed another latent failure.

Case Study #10: Ten times the prescribed amount of insulin is administered.
The setting is a long-term care unit. An elderly patient with diabetes has stumbled and x-ray confirms a luxation of his hip prosthesis. During the evening the orthopedic surgeon makes an unsuccessful attempt under anesthesia to reduce the luxation. The surgeon orders the patient to be prepared for surgery for the next morning and the patient is transferred back to the long-term care unit.

The night nurse in the long-term care unit has very little experience in preparing patients for surgery. She tries to carry out the surgeon's orders, which are stated in very general terms and refer to numerous vaguely worded procedures. The nurse finds these procedures difficult to understand and they are apparently very outdated.

She has to make several phone calls to physicians and staff to ask questions about what to do. Among other issues, she is very confused about the insulin infusion she has to prepare for the patient. When she finally calculates the dose of insulin, she commits an error and administers 10 times too much insulin. The medication error was not detected until the caregivers in the postanesthesia care unit had a difficult time awakening the patient. After checking the blood glucose level, which was very low, glucose was administered, the patient recovered, and the accident had a happy ending (for the patient, not the nurse).

Accident Analysis: The active failure was committed by the nurse. How the nurse could commit this insulin-dosing error was obviously due to her mental overload. She had to use knowledge-based problem solving for a problem she rarely had to solve, and she had been given insufficient instructions. Listed below are the factors that contributed to this inappropriate problem-solving environment for the nurse, thus triggering the active failure and causing the system to lose control.

- The procedural instructions available to her were outdated and poorly written.
- It was not suitable for the doctor to write a general prescription for insulin in this situation, leaving the burden of interpretation and calculation to the nurse.
- No preoperative assessment was done by the anesthesiologist. The argument was (wrongly) given that the patient had only a few hours earlier received general anesthesia and therefore did not need another assessment.
- It might have been more appropriate to admit the patient temporally to the orthopedic ward following the first procedure. The staff in this unit are well trained in preparing patients for surgery.

The *latent failures* in this case can thus be summarized as follows:

- Poor document control allowed procedures to be poorly written and become outdated.
- Poor process control existed at the following points:
  —Prescriptions should be written in specific terms for all patients.
  —Preoperative assessment should always be done.
- Interdepartmental coordination was poor.

Situational factors were the unlucky combination of the patient's being in the long-term care unit and general anesthesia having been given to the patient earlier in the same 24-hour period. Another situational factor was that in this long-term care unit only insulin pens are used; thus the nurse had a poor mental frame of reference for the proper volume of fluid to expect to see in a syringe. Had the same active failure happened at a department where syringes were also in use, the nurse might have had a better chance of visually detecting her error immediately.

Procedures demanding double-checks of insulin dosage calculations or computerized calculation aids are safety barriers that could have caught the nurse's active failure before patient harm occurred. However, these safety barriers were not in place at the time of the accident.

Case Study #11: Patient with sepsis is discharged without antibiotics.

The setting is a general surgical ward. The patient has been admitted because of blood loss anemia. During the stay the patient gets a high fever, a sepsis is diagnosed, and he is treated with antibiotics. After a week in the hospital the cause of the blood loss has not yet been found; however, the patient declares that he wants to go home immediately and is discharged. The investigation for the cause of the anemia is planned to continue in the outpatient department. A few days after discharge, the patient is admitted with fever and heart failure. Now it is detected that he was discharged from the hospital without antibiotics. He has to undergo major thoracic surgery to treat an abscess on his aortic valve prosthesis.

Accident Analysis: The *active failure* was committed by a junior doctor who forgot to prescribe antibiotics at the time the patient was discharged. However, the accident analysis showed that the antibiotics had been inadvertently stopped the day before (Sunday) without anybody at morning rounds on the day of discharge (Monday) noticing this oversight.

Several *situational factors* were found to exist. This event occurred during a summer holiday period and the whole team of doctors on Monday were back fresh from vacation while the previous team went on vacation the preceding Friday. The senior physician on duty during the weekend was a stand-in from another unit and her time was filled attending to acute problems.

The *latent failures* included rather dangerous procedures for medication prescription during weekends. The decision-making culture at morning rounds was also viewed as a latent failure. The doctors obtain the information necessary for decision making by allowing the nurse to give an oral résumé of cases rather than reading themselves what is recorded in patient charts. In this case the nurse told the doctors what she found important; namely, that the focus for the patient's bleeding had not yet been found and that the patient was fed up with being in the hospital. If the doctors had read the patient's chart, they would have seen a clear narrative of the sepsis and that the patient had had an aortic valve replacement. Further analysis showed that the allocation of responsibilities among the physicians on the team were ill defined, and this was also felt to contribute to the accident. The latent failures could be summarized like this:

- Inappropriate routines for decision making at rounds
- Inappropriate planning of vacations (one team member should overlap)
- Indistinct allocation of responsibility among team members

Case #10 and case #11 illustrate how easy it is to find a culprit to blame (the nurse and the junior physician). But when the case is analyzed, it becomes obvious that these individuals had inherited the effect of several latent failures. They had the bad luck of being at the wrong place at the wrong time. However, if the latent failures had not been actively looked for, they probably would not have been discovered. Thus the information necessary for taking appropriate preventive actions would not have been obtained.

FRAMEWORK FOR INVESTIGATING MEDICAL ACCIDENTS

Whether a safe system can be designed based on knowledge of previous medical mistakes remains open to debate. Authors arguing against this assumption claim that the same accident will never happen again because the combination of situational factors and latent failures is unique and will almost certainly never combine in the same way again. They are partly right. The same situational factors that triggered the latent failures in the cases described in the last section might not occur again. But many of the latent failures identified are not unique to these accidents. The latent failures endanger system stability in other circumstances that present with other unforeseen situational factors. Therefore, it is worthwhile to track them down.

The aim of investigating a medical accident is to obtain information about how the system lost control so that preventive actions can be taken to improve the future safety and reliability of the system. The interaction between system-controlling components and situational factors is complex, and a considerable amount of information must be gathered during an accident investigation. Thus, some sort of method for structuring and analyzing information is very important. The method should also be fairly simple and easy to understand for the staff and the organization. It must be an aid, not a hindrance, to the investigation.

These requirements are fulfilled by the MTO analysis method. As mentioned early in the chapter, the acronym MTO stands for Man-Technique-Organization. It exists under different names such as HPES (Human Performance Enhancement System) and ASSET.[14] It was adopted by the Swedish nuclear power industry and we have now adapted and applied it to health care accidents. The steps of an MTO analysis are listed in figure 3-3. Each of these steps is described in subsequent sections.[15]

MTO analysis (or a similar analysis) ought to be done following serious medical mistakes or sentinel events. These accidents seldom occur

Figure 3-3.   Steps of the MTO Analysis

- Develop a preliminary map of the event.
- Conduct a preliminary cause analysis.
- Conduct on-site investigation and interviews.
- Review event mapping.
- Review cause analysis.
- Conduct barrier analysis.
- Identify situational factors.
- Identify latent failures.
- Identify absent or insufficient safety barriers.
- Develop an agenda for preventive actions.

because of a single error. Normally, several latent failures interact in a system with poor defenses (flawed safety barriers), and the latent failures are not found unless systematically looked for. MTO analysis can also be of use in examining more complicated near accidents with several operators involved. MTO analysis is not a cost-effective choice for investigating fairly simple incidents.

MTO Teams

The MTO analysis should ideally be conducted by a team of people from the health care organization where the accident occurred. Because of the personal involvement of team members, investigation findings are more likely to result in organizational changes, contrary to what happens if an external expert supplies all the answers. The MTO analysis team must receive sufficient introduction to the investigation method and ongoing support throughout the process. I have tested different training and support approaches and have found the model illustrated in figure 3-4 to be most effective. Of crucial importance to the MTO team is management's backing. Organizational leaders should view the MTO analysis as an important trigger for improvement processes.

Because error management is a cross-scientific problem, the team members should have basic working knowledge in the following fields:

- Cognitive psychology
- Systems theory
- Process reengineering

Figure 3-4. Training and Support of the Team in MTO Analysis

- The team is introduced to the MTO analysis method. This session lasts for up to one day. During the introduction they practice the method on a case study. This training is conducted by an external MTO analysis expert, but it could be conducted by an internal expert if such a person exists in the organization.
- The MTO analysis expert helps the team with the preliminary MTO analysis.
- The team does the on-site investigation and the review of the analysis. The MTO analysis expert stands by as "sparring partner" for the team when needed.
- The MTO analysis expert is involved in the final analysis before the team writes the report.

- Quality systems audit
- MTO methodology

Team members must be medical professionals (physicians and nurses) but not necessarily specialists in the same discipline in which the accident took place. I think team members are best recruited from senior physicians and nurses, but should not be so senior that the minds have lost their alertness. A suitable size for a team at a medium-sized hospital could be four members.

The team members also need to have certain personal qualifications. They must, of course, have a genuine interest in error management. They must have a high personal integrity. They should have a good ability to think in process and system terms (not so common among physicians) and be analytical. They must be empathic, be good listeners, and conduct themselves with dignity and respect for both the complexity of their task and the poor operators involved in the accident. They must be flexible and able to adapt easily to new information (not getting stuck in their own prejudices).

It might be realistic to establish such a team as a standing committee in a hospital or for a chain of hospitals. Or it may be preferable to form ad hoc teams that are charged with investigating one specific accident. Whatever model is chosen, the teams should be organizationally aligned under administration, perhaps in the quality management or risk management department.

Establishing an MTO team takes quite some effort in both member selection and training. In my experience, training of a standing MTO team could be done in two to three days, depending on team members' previous experience. In some of my classes we have used a half-day for a theoretical introduction and the rest of the time in hands-on investigation training using real cases provided by the students. Ad hoc MTO teams established for one particular accident are provided abbreviated training. Two to three hours are devoted to a basic introduction, and then the team takes over the investigation (I've already done a preliminary analysis). After the initial training, the MTO expert need only meet two or three times with the team during an accident investigation to check the progress of the analysis and sort out methodological problems.

Gather Information   The MTO analysis team begins the investigation process by reviewing the written reports of the accident that were completed by involved staff. These reports should have been completed as soon as possible after the accident occurred. "Involved staff" are defined as those who committed an active failure and those otherwise involved in the actual situation of care; that is, the involved team. Included are also the closest superiors to involved staff and, finally, heads of relevant departments (for example, chief of surgery, nursing director, and so on).

A crucial part of information gathering are interviews conducted with relevant people in the organization, as it is unlikely they wrote down everything that the MTO analysis team might need. These interviews also provide a golden opportunity for the MTO analysis team to enter into fruitful dialogues with operators and management, thus improving their understanding of the human-system misfits that contributed to the accident. This part of the analysis must be carefully conducted. If the involved staff and/or management are not already members of the MTO analysis team, they may be nervous and insecure when discussing the events surrounding the incidents. Whether these interviews are done individually by members of the MTO team or as a team activity (people are asked to attend one or more team meetings), the following points should be considered:

- Be well prepared.
- Always make an appointment.
- Never go behind the back of department management.
- Be very clear and specific as to the aim of the investigation.
- Do not schedule interviews too tightly (one hour per interview is a good guideline).
- Create a relaxed atmosphere; begin with small talk.
- Start the interview with an open mind.
- Skip the tape recorder; make notes instead.
- Interview as a rule only one person at a time, but allow a colleague to be present if the person being interviewed so desires.

The team uses the information gathered in written reports and oral interviews to construct an MTO analysis diagram. This process flow diagram is the tool used for structuring the analysis. An example of an MTO analysis diagram that has yet to be filled in with accident investigation data is shown in table 3-1. This diagram can be handdrawn or computer generated using spreadsheet software. In the cells across the top of the diagram, the chain of events that took place during the accident are noted. This table has four columns with cells for four events. The finished product will have as many columns as the number of events in the event chain.

The factors to be analyzed are listed down the left side of the table (one per row). In the MTO analyses I have conducted, a minimum of four factors are analyzed: contributing causes, situational factors, safety barriers, and latent failures. More factors can naturally be added at the discretion of the investigator. For research purposes, I often add another separate row for noting "cognitive failure mechanisms." For a discussion of these failure mechanisms, see the section earlier in this chapter on how humans solve problems and why errors occur.

As can be seen from the diagram, the row for "contributing causes" on the MTO analysis table serves a double function as denoted by the label "questions/contributing causes." During the investigation a lot of questions come to the minds of the team members; for example, "How could this happen?" or "Why did she do it like this?" These questions are noted in this row and then, when they are resolved during the personal interviews, the answers turn into direct causes.

Map the Event The events leading up to the adverse occurrence are listed on the MTO analysis table in sequential order in the cells along the top. This event mapping should be as precise as possible. The chronology is important so dates and, if known, the hour and minute of the event should be recorded (hour and minute are not necessary if the event extends over several days). Event mapping requires some experience.

Table 3-1. Example of a Blank MTO Diagram

Date/time				
Event				
Questions/ contributing causes				
Situational factors				
Safety barriers				
Latent failures				

Note: The diagram headings can be designed to the taste and need of the analyst.

The most common error is to include too many actions in each cell. Only one step in the sequence of events should be stated per cell or the MTO analysis team will get into trouble during the cause analysis phase; that is, if you squeeze a sequence that actually comprises three separate actions into one cell in the event mapping, then you might find that you end up with three different causes for these actions, thus breaking the rule of "one cell-one cause" in the cause analysis.

Another common fault is to start the analysis too late in the sequence, thus missing important situational factors. For example, if the accident takes place in the emergency department, do not necessarily confine the analysis to this unit. Maybe the investigation should start a couple of days earlier when the patient got the first symptoms of the illness, or at least include the action where the patient calls an ambulance. The end-point for the investigation is easier to define than the start-point. If the accident causes a patient death, this is the end-point. If not, corrective actions taken after the accident should be included in the analysis.

Identify Active Failures   After the team is satisfied that the events leading up to the accident are clearly understood and documented, the next step is to identify which events represent active failures. You may recall from the previous section that active failures are considered to be errors made by the operators performing the processes. This inquiry should not be conducted until personal interviews have been completed; otherwise information necessary to give the team a complete picture of the problem won't be available.

It is not always easy for the team to determine what is a right or wrong action. It may be necessary to ask a neutral observer, perhaps someone from another facility or another unit who has the same educational background, experience, and work tasks as the operator whose action is to be assessed. Ask this neutral observer, "In a similar situation, with similar preconditions, what should have been done?"

Identify Contributing Causes and Situational Factors   In those vertical columns of table 3-1 considered to represent an active failure, the team identifies contributing causes for this failure. A contributing cause represents the most immediate or obvious reason for the active failure.[16] More than one contributing cause may be present for each active failure. To aid the team in identifying contributing causes, a taxonomy covering the major causes of medical mistakes has been developed. The taxonomy, shown in table 3-2, is a simplified version of the HPES (nuclear power model MTO analysis). This taxonomy is also useful for the team to have available during personal interviews to ensure that all relevant questions are asked of involved staff and management.

Situational factors are defined as unforeseen circumstances that play a major part in the evolution of the accident. It is often these unlucky circumstances that can explain why the process went wrong this one time even though the process was carried through in the usual way. These situational factors are also mapped on table 3-1.

The contributing cause(s) and situational factor(s) are noted in the cells immediately below the relevant active failure. The team may be tempted to stop the investigation at this stage, thinking that if the contributing causes are fixed, the system can be returned to a stable state. However, it is important to complete the MTO analysis model or otherwise the latent failures won't be identified. As we have seen, a medical accident is caused by a unique combination and interaction of several system-controlling components (among other totally unforeseen situational factors), and these will probably not combine in this way for many years to come. Thus, elimination of identified contributing causes might only be a safeguard against a similar accident, not a cure.

A superficial analysis can also give a counterproductive effect. More procedures might be written, more operators might be instructed to comply with double-checks, vigorous ad hoc training programs might be undertaken, and the administrative control concerning adherence to instructions might be tightened up.[17] The overall effect of this superficial analysis might be that instead of getting a safer system, one gets a fuzzier and more awkward system that is less reliable than the old one. This can be avoided by doing a proper MTO analysis. The cause-effect chain should be traced so far backward that eventual deficiencies in the quality system can be disclosed. Improvements in the quality system, as a result of an MTO analysis, will have an overall beneficial effect on system reliability instead of only preventing an accident that will anyhow (almost) never happen again.

Identify Ineffective Safety Barriers and Latent Failures   Next, the team identifies the safety barriers that were in place at the time of the accident and the latent failures. Most health care processes have built-in safeguards to prevent errors from reaching the patient. The MTO analysis

Table 3-2.   Taxonomy of Contributing Causes

Cause Categories	Examples of Problems in this Category
Oral communication	• Oral communication from the sender is imprecise. • Receiver does not acknowledge the message. • Standardized vocabulary is not used. • Unnecessary talk is not avoided. • The sender and receiver did not "tune in" to each other (this takes a longer time if they are not already acquainted with one another).
Written procedures	• The information in the procedure is given in the wrong sequence, or a sequence has been omitted. • The text is difficult to understand, ambiguous, or too elaborate. • The readability is poor (sentences too long, poor layout). • The procedure mixes target groups. • The procedure is written for both experienced and inexperienced users. • Too many people are instructed to do the same thing, and therefore nobody does it. • The available instruction is outdated or otherwise invalid. • It is not clear for which situation the procedure should be used. • It is not clear who should use the procedure.
Workplace design/physical environment	• Maneuver gear or display is badly designed, hard to reach, or hard to read. • Readability for important information is bad. • Acoustical signals are inappropriately designed. • Workplace design is inappropriate. • Equipment is badly situated. • There are too many people. • Lighting is insufficient. • Distracting noise is present.
Working environment	• There is insufficient time for staff to prepare for work assignments. • Not enough staff are allocated to work tasks or they are insufficiently trained for tasks. • Planning of activities is not coordinated between departments. • Staff members are easily distracted when performing simultaneous tasks.
Task supervision	• Tasks are not properly defined for the operator. • There is insufficient follow-up from the supervisor (e.g., staff do not report when they are in trouble or when task is done). • The level of training necessary to perform the task is not defined. • Staff performance assessments are not done.
Training	• Training of operator is insufficient. • There is insufficient repetition of training. • Educational goals are missing or goals are not related to the task. • No follow-up assessment of educational effect is done.

team will want to identify the technical and/or administrative barriers that failed to prevent the mistake under investigation. Latent failures are those circumstances that trapped the operator into committing an active failure, impeded error detection, or created a messy situation that negatively influenced the operator's performance and that can be considered flaws in the organization's system for quality management. As described earlier in this chapter, latent failures are attributed to the people who influence the system but who are not active participants; for example, housekeeping, maintenance, information systems, and management.

The team identifies missing safety barriers and latent failures by asking the following questions about each active failure:

- Which safety barriers, if any, failed to stop the error from reaching the patient?
- Could any safety barrier have been built into the system at this point so as to hinder the operator making this error?
- Could a safety barrier be designed in such a way that the error could be detected before harmful system influence took place?
- Can a latent failure be identified that:
  —trapped the operator into making this error?
  —delayed or prevented the error from being detected?
  —created a disorderly environment that may have activated the error?

Safety barriers and latent failures are entered into the appropriate cells on the MTO diagram. Since accident evolution is often very complex, the team may find that it is sometimes difficult to fit safety barriers and latent failures into the time chronology; that is, in the same column where the active failure is mapped. For example, in the insulin overdose case (case #10 described on page 116), the causes for the nurse's active failure really came into play long before the active failure was committed. Also, the same latent failure can play a role at several points during the chain of events. Simply map it the first time it discloses itself and repeatedly map it on the diagram for each occasion that the same failure exerts system influence.

A schematic example of an excerpt from an MTO analysis for an incident involving delayed diagnosis of appendicitis is shown in table 3-3. Along the top row are the actions or events that took place in

Table 3-3. Example of a Schematic Diagram from an MTO Analysis

	A	B	C	D	E	F
1	Date/time	May 5 18:00	May 5 19:00	May 5 20:00	May 1 22:00	May 3 15:00
2	Event	Patient has had stomach pain for two days, temp of 38° C., nausea.	Patient calls ED and is told to come in for an examination.	Patient examined by physician, who diagnoses gastritis.	Patient sent home with instructions to return if condition gets worse.	Patient returns in ambulance in preshock due to peritonitis from ruptured appendix.
3	Contributing causes			Resident physician inexperienced		
4	Situational factors			Slight improvement of patient during stay in ED		
5	Safety barriers			The standard operating procedure is for the resident physician to call senior surgeon to examine patients with abdominal pain before patient leaves hospital.		
6	Latent failures			Proper training for resident physicians' work tasks not defined		

chronological order. In this example, action D ("misdiagnosis") was an erroneous action. One contributing cause was identified ("inexperienced physician"). One situational factor ("patient appeared to improve") was found and a safety barrier ("senior surgeon was supposed to examine patient") was identified that might either have prevented the erroneous action or the harmful influence on the system caused by the erroneous action. The contributing cause was eventually traced to a latent failure in the training system ("no mechanism in place to communicate 'standard operating procedures' to resident physicians"). An actual MTO analysis diagram can be five to ten pages in length.

Acting on the MTO Analysis Results

The knowledge from the analysis must be put to use in order to improve system safety; otherwise the exercise is a waste of time and money. The improvement action plan should be developed after internal discussions with the "process owners" in the facility. The people directly involved in the processes often have a very good understanding of system risks and are best positioned to recommend necessary changes. Once the action plans have been determined, add the subtasks that must be done along with deadlines and assigned responsibilities.

More often than not the number of disclosed latent failures and absent safety barriers are greater than can be remedied at once. It may become necessary to prioritize where improvements will be made. The criteria to be considered when setting priorities includes the frequency of process disturbances caused by the latent failure and the severity of the disturbance. Since quantitative data concerning process disturbances are scarce in health care it may be necessary to estimate the frequency. Latent failures with little potential for losing system control can nevertheless produce frequent minor disturbances. This in itself can be a reason to give it high priority for remedial action because it can cost the organization a lot of money for the rework and corrective actions that may be necessary. It should be borne in mind that latent failures can interact in a nasty way so that a number of less potentially harmful latent failures may some day mess up a process, thus creating a dangerous situation with loss of system control.

A latent failure with potential for very harmful system effects can sometimes be very expensive or difficult to remedy. An alternative is to circumvent the failure by designing strong safety barriers that catch the effect of the active failure caused by this latent failure.

THE ROLE OF MTO ANALYSIS IN ERROR MANAGEMENT

Reason suggests that organizational *error management* must be proactive as well as reactive to be successful at containing and reducing error.[18] MTO analysis is primarily a reactive error containment tool. Health care systems cannot rely solely on what is learned in the analysis of yesterday's mistakes in order to design safer systems. Reactive investigations must be supplemented by proactive error reduction activities. Discussed below are the drawbacks to using MTO analysis (and other accident investigation techniques) as the only element in an organization error management program.

In an MTO analysis, the accident chooses which processes will be analyzed, and these may not be the riskiest processes in the organization. Since situational factors are innumerable and the number of combinations of latent failures and insufficient safety barriers is immense, an organization will have to wait for accidents for many years before all processes are closely examined. This will of course be extremely costly and unethical too because many patients must be killed or hurt to "produce" the accidents.

Such a strategy would not work anyway because an organization is never stable; it is always changing due to a lot of different reasons. Therefore, the belief that better system reliability can be achieved by acting only on information from yesterday's mistakes is about as realistic as the likelihood that Sisyphus should succeed with his task of getting the stone to the top of the hill.

MTO analysis should be used to learn as much as possible from occurred accidents. To improve process reliability, another, proactive approach should be used to keep ahead of the accident. Several proactive methods have been described and applied to complex technical systems,[19] but thus far there is no tradition for the application of such a method in health care. Researchers at the Lund Institute of Technology in Sweden have developed and applied a method in health care which we call DEB analysis (the acronym stands for Disturbance-Effect-Barrier).

The principle is much the same as MTO analysis, but because no accident has occurred there is no event to map. Instead, a *process* in the organization is chosen for study. The DEB analysis can be summarized like this:

- Choose a process to study.
- Form an analysis team.
- Map the process carefully.
- Hypothesize disturbances.
- Validate hypotheses by observation, interview, or incident reports (if available).
- Evaluate system effect of validated disturbances.
- Look for latent failures and safety barriers that need to be developed/redesigned.
- Identify and implement error containment action plans.

The possible system effect of the disturbance is evaluated, latent failures that make the error possible are identified, and possible safety barriers that might be able to prevent harmful system effect of the error are looked for. The next section briefly describes the application of the DEB analysis method in a department of oncology at a university hospital.

DEB Analysis Case Study

To conduct this DEB analysis, two support analysts spent approximately five working days each in gathering the necessary data. This included process mapping and validation of hypotheses on process disturbances. Another two days were spent on report preparation on completion of the project.

Choose a Process to Study The chosen process was the treatment of a patient with cytotoxic agents within one unit.

Form an Analysis Team A group from the ward unit was established, consisting of two nurses (one of these was the head nurse for the unit) and a physician (oncologist) who had shown interest in the project. The group also included a pharmacist, who was supervisor for the cytotoxic agent preparation unit at the hospital pharmacy.

Map the Process Carefully Because the chosen process was far more complicated than anticipated, the steps divided into the following subprocesses:

- Decision on treating a patient with cytotoxic agents
- Planning for treatment (when the patient arrives on the unit)
- Prescription (preparing the cytotoxic agent treatment chart [CAC])
- Preparation (at the pharmacy)
- Administering drugs to the patient
- Follow-up of ongoing treatment
- Planning for next treatment cycle

The whole process, including all the components in the subprocesses, were mapped in a diagram resembling the MTO diagram.

Hypothesize Disturbances A number of hypotheses concerning possible disturbances in the process were generated. To perform this step, the team asked the following questions about each step in the process: What happens if we influence the process at this step too much? too little? wrongly? not at all?

Validate Disturbances The hypothetical answers to the questions in the preceding step were validated by interviewing the process owners to determine if these disturbances could actually happen or have happened.

Evaluate System Effect of Validated Disturbances In this step, possible consequences for negative impact on system stability were assessed; that is, what was the probability that a certain disturbance could create a system failure (serious accident) or only a minor process aberration? This step is closely integrated with the next step. The probability for a certain disturbance to cause system failure is of course much higher if no efficient safety barriers exist to counteract the harmful system influence of a disturbance.

Look for Latent Failures and Safety Barriers That Need to Be Developed/ Redesigned At this stage in the DEB analysis we are able to identify some major dangers in the system. One danger was that the most frequent, and the most serious, disturbances took place during the doctor's prescription on the CAC. For the most part, other types of prescription errors were regularly caught and remedied by the pharmacy preparation unit; however, CAC prescription errors tended to be missed. If the physician mixes up regimes and chooses the wrong one or misunderstands the dosage guidelines, this error (illustrated as a disturbance arrow on the diagram) had a high probability of shooting through the whole system without getting caught before it hit the patient.

The oncology nurse served as a safety barrier for CAC prescription-writing errors (the last possible one before the error hit the patient); however, this barrier appeared to have flaws. The CAC was often very poorly written, making it difficult for the nurse to act as a safety barrier. Further, the CAC layout was inappropriate, making it difficult for the nurse to get an overview of the day's medications. The nurse-safety barrier might work with experienced nurses but would be weakened with inexperienced nurses who may be unwilling to question a physician's prescription.

The group was also not happy to find that the nurse-safety barrier was an informal one (checking the correctness of the CAC was not a defined responsibility of the nurse). The nurses took on a responsibility that they had not been formally delegated to perform. This lack of formalization was a problem, too, concerning the interaction between the pharmacy chemotherapy preparation staff and the unit. The pharmacy staff did a lot of quality control of CAC content. Such checking was not a task formally delegated to the pharmacy unit, although it had been going on for quite some time. This might lead to a dangerous situation in which the physicians begin to rely on pharmacy double-checks only to find that they are not taking place.

All in all, the DEB analysis disclosed 12 latent system failures and 6 flawed safety barriers, all with the potential of killing or seriously harming the patient on that day in the future when bad luck occurs.

Identify and Implement Error Containment Action Plans The final DEB analysis report recommended several actions plans, including the following:

- Introduction of computer-aided prescriptions for the CAC
- Recommendations that responsibilities be clarified between the different actors in the system
- Implementation of double-checks on important decisions

- Standardization of equipment (infusion pumps) in cooperating ward units
- Introduction of proper feedback loops concerning handling of blood tests

Because an incident-reporting system was not in place in this unit prior to the DEB analysis, it was very difficult for the group to quantify the study findings. Recommendations were made to put such a reporting system in place.

CONCLUSION

Accidents in health care are a matter of considerable concern, and the extent of such accidents might be substantial. Surprisingly few studies have been done to shed light on this sinister area of medical care. One extensive study was done by Brennan and others—the Harvard Medical Practice Study.[20] According to this study, medical accidents occur in 3 percent of admissions, and some of these might result in damage or death to a patient. When the results from this study are applied to a country like Sweden (where there is no reason to believe the safety of medical care to be worse or better than in the United States) with 8 million inhabitants, health care appears to be more dangerous than road traffic.

Risk management in areas where great disasters have occurred (nuclear power, air and rail traffic, shipping) has made tremendous advances during the past decade in understanding accident behavior in complex technical systems. Unfortunately, investigations of medical accidents are still largely a matter of finding and punishing the humans involved. This obsolete approach to medical accident investigations has serious negative effects:

- Many staff members, accused of having caused an accident, feel guilt and shame during the rest of their professional career, and this may have a negative effect on their future ability as problem solvers.
- The root causes of the accidents are not identified, thus impeding the development of preventive measures.

- Litigation is costly and the money could have been spent more productively on proper preventive actions.

Health care production takes place in what can be called a complex system. Risk or error management in complex technical systems has made tremendous advances during the past two decades but has thus far been applied only to a limited extent to health care, though health care also is a complex system. The modern way of looking at accidents suggests that they basically result from interface problems between human and system.

The term *human error* is controversial because it contains a great amount of hindsight judgment; a faulty action can result in disaster or nothing happens, depending on circumstances and good luck. But both actions were nevertheless erroneous, or weren't they? The mechanisms causing human error can be understood from models in the field of cognitive psychology concerning our problem-solving strategies. Our memory database is the long-term memory, which has seemingly unlimited capacity for storing information and it works outside our conscious control. The working memory, on the contrary, is the conscious part of our thinking. It has a very limited capacity and quickly gets overloaded. It is the working memory that directs our attention toward important parts of a problem. By applying this knowledge concerning cognitive strategies, accident investigators can recognize how latent system failures exert negative influence on the caregiver's problem-solving capacity.

It is important to analyze system behavior in medical accidents. The system failures leading up to the event can be subdivided as active and latent failures. Active failures are those committed by the operators. Latent failures (or root causes) are flaws in the management system of the organization. Latent failures are mostly activated by situational factors, which are unforeseen, unlucky circumstances. Latent failures trap operators into committing active failures, impede error detection, or create messy situations. Unless the system has good safety barriers to absorb the harmful system effect of the active failures, loss of system control becomes imminent.

Latent failures and flawed safety barriers must be actively investigated after an accident; otherwise they are easily missed. A framework for accident analysis of medical accidents was presented under the name of MTO analysis. It is a concept originally developed by NASA, later adopted by the nuclear power industry, and now adapted to health care. In the MTO analysis the chain of events leading to an accident is carefully mapped. Contributing causes, situational factors, latent failures, and deficient safety barriers are looked for in a systematic way.

A safe and reliable system for tomorrow cannot be based solely on analyses of yesterday's mistakes. Therefore, a proactive method for reliability analyses of processes in health care was presented (DEB analysis) together with a case study of its application. By studying the negative effects that human operators may exert on the system and the system's ability to absorb these negative effects, a "forgiving system" can be designed. Such a system will maintain its stability better than a nonforgiving system. It is imperative that health care systems be designed in a forgiving way to minimize the risk of medical mistakes and patient injury.

References and Note

1. H. Van Cott. "Human Errors: Their Causes and Reduction," in S. Bogner, ed., *Human Error in Medicine* (Hillsdale, NJ: Lawrence Erlbaum Associates, 1994).

2. V. Chopra et al. "Reported Significant Observations During Anesthesia: A Prospective Analysis Over an 18-Month Period," *British Journal of Anesthesia* 68 (1992): 13–17.

3. J. B. Cooper et al. "Preventable Anesthesia Mishaps: A Study of Human Factors," *Anesthesiology* 49 (1978): 399–406.

4. The examples included in this chapter are derived from the medical accident files of the Swedish National Board of Health and Welfare.

5. J. T. Reason. *Human Error: Causes and Consequences* (New York: Cambridge University Press, 1990).

6. Ibid.

7. Ibid.

8. R. I. Cook and D. D. Woods. "Operating at the Sharp End: The Complexity of Human Error," in S. Bogner, ed., *Human Error in Medicine* (Hillsdale, NJ: Lawrence Erlbaum Associates, 1994).

9. J. Rasmussen. "Human Errors: A Taxonomy for Describing Human Malfunction in Industrial Installations," *Journal of Occupational Accidents* 4 (1982): 311–33.

10. Ibid.

11. H. VanCott. "Human Errors."

12. J. T. Reason. *Human Error.*

13. D. W. Bates et al. "Effect of Computerized Physician Order Entry and a Team Intervention on Prevention of Serious Medication Errors," *JAMA* 280, no. 15 (1998): 1311–16.

14. ASSET guidelines. IAEA-tecdoc-573, IAEA, Wienna (1990).

15. It should be noted that the MTO analysis steps used by the National Board of Health and Welfare in Sweden are slightly different from those discussed in this chapter. The Board of Health investigates all medical accidents and a representative from the board serves as the expert on the MTO analysis team. Most medical accident investigations in the United States are conducted internally by the involved organization, and people from outside the organization rarely sit on the analysis team. The MTO analysis model presented in this chapter has been adapted to fit the circumstances most often found in U.S. medical accident investigations.

16. P. E. Wilson, L. D. Dell, and G. F. Anderson. *Root Cause Analysis: A Tool for Total Quality Management* (Milwaukee, WI: ASQ Quality Press, 1993), p. 10.

17. J. Rasmussen. "What Can be Learned from Human Error Reports?" in K. Duncan, M. Gruneberg, and D. Wallis, eds., *Changes in Working Life* (London, Eng.: John Wiley and Sons, 1980).

18. J. Reason. *Managing the Risks of Organizational Accidents* (Aldershot, Eng.: Ashgate Publishing, Ltd., 1997), p. 125.

19. L. Harms-Ringdahl. *Safety Analysis: Principles and Practice in Occupational Safety* (London, Eng.: Elsevier Applied Science, 1993).

20. T .A. Brennan et al. "Incidence of Adverse Events and Negligence in Hospitalized Patients: Results from the Harvard Medical Practice Study I," *New England Journal of Medicine* 324 (1991): 370–76.

4

Accident Investigation and Anticipatory Failure Analysis in Hospitals

Sanford E. Feldman, MD, FACS
Douglas W. Roblin, PhD

During the past 20 years, studies have shown that approximately 5 percent of hospitalized patients are injured during the course of their treatment.[1,2] Many of these injuries may have been preventable. Nearly one-fifth of the injuries are the result of egregious errors committed during the course of seemingly routine care—such as administration of a gross overdose or a fatal wrong medication.[3] Although more patients are now being cared for in outpatient facilities, the majority of reported medical accidents occur in hospitals. Like petrochemical plants or airlines, hospitals can be considered "hazard systems."[4] A hazard is a "physical situation with a potential for human injury, damage to property, damage to the environment, or some combination of these."

Current health care quality appraisal methods too often focus on clinician error as a principal causal factor contributing to patient injury. Inquiry has been generally concerned with issues of negligence or incompetence; corrective action may lead to remedial professional education, mentoring, or, rarely, sanction. Those injuries that are not attributed to clinician error may often be dismissed as random events that are not likely to recur.

Recently, hospitals have been encouraged by the Joint Commission on Accreditation of Healthcare Organizations to use methods employed in private industry for investigating the cause of adverse events. These accident investigation methods, including root cause analysis, can aid caregivers in identifying the underlying system faults that allowed the clinical error to occur in the first place.[5] Isolating and correcting root causes can diminish the risk of recurrence of similar patient injuries. Current approaches to hospital quality appraisal focus on the immediately obvious clinician error but rarely pursue investigation of the causal influence of latent system faults. Latent system faults in the hospital include error in design or maintenance of medical equipment, defects in information management, and failure in the training of physicians or other staff in work processes.

There are many different methods of root cause analysis, several of which are described in this book. Regardless of the terminology used to portray the process, all methods place emphasis on finding changes in the system that might be effective in reducing accident risk.

An effective patient safety initiative should include both strategies for retrospective analysis of an accident to determine "what went wrong" and strategies for prospective analysis of operations to determine what might go wrong. Such strategies involve comprehensive, ongoing study of the following:

- Each accident to identify and clarify the relationship between active human error and latent system faults
- Near-miss circumstances in which a catastrophic accident was averted but lessons about accident evolution might still be learned
- Industrial organization and work processes in anticipation of the possibility of accident occurrence

Discussion in this chapter is directed toward those individuals in a hospital who currently review iatrogenic injuries to patients. These include physicians, quality and risk management staff, plant safety personnel, and other individuals who are involved in the design, operation, and review of safe hospital practices. The objectives of this chapter are to provide an overview of accident analysis and implementation of sustained inquiry in support of ongoing patient safety advocacy. The application of root cause analysis to the investigation of injuries to hospitalized patients is discussed. Two examples of actual cases are described to illustrate how active errors and latent system faults can be isolated. Finally, some recommendations for a sustained hospital patient safety enhancement program are outlined. This program would include ongoing retrospective analyses of patient injuries, collection and evaluation of near-miss events, and assessment of various hospital functions to isolate the latent system faults that represent accidents waiting to happen.

ACCIDENT INVESTIGATION

Industries such as petrochemical processing, nuclear power generation, and air transportation are complex sociotechnical systems involving the coordination of many diverse human and mechanical elements. Many of these industries have established reputations for high reliability and have achieved outstanding records for safe operation.[6,7] Yet in many of these enterprises, accidents inevitably occur.[8] Accidents are injury-causing events that occur unexpectedly and unintentionally.[9,10] Investigation of accidents in manufacturing and transportation has led to the recognition that serious accidents cannot be explained simply as a consequence of operator or pilot error. Awareness of the contribution of faults latent in the industrial systems (equipment design or maintenance, organization and management of work processes, conflicting or ambiguous production goals) has grown with each succeeding study of a catastrophic accident.

An accident investigation is undertaken to isolate root causes that increased the risk that an accident would occur and to assess whether the organization might have had some control over the circumstances that led to the evolution of that accident. A framework for isolating root causes includes identification of the following:

- The sequence of events contributing to the accident
- Events within that sequence that represent active errors
- Points in the sequence that represent latent system faults

In chapter 3 of this book, Dr. Sven Ternov provided a comprehensive discussion of the causes of human errors and how those errors contribute to accidents. That subject will not be reiterated in this chapter; however, a few basic reminders about the difference between active errors and latent system faults are offered below.

Active Errors and Latent System Faults

Because humans are fallible, active errors—slips, mistakes, unsafe practices—occur in the course of routine, normal production processes in complex sociotechnical systems.[11-13] Slips are unintended deviations from an intended plan, often due to distractions and inattention. Mistakes represent poor judgment, incorrect inference, or faulty reasoning in the conduct of an intended plan of action. Unsafe practices or rule violations are conscious decisions to proceed in circumstances where adverse risks are known. Uncertainty, confusion, distraction, and urgency to "do the right thing" facilitate these errors. Active errors have an immediate impact on system state and function. Their immediacy and proximity make them conspicuous events in the evolution of an accident.

Latent system faults are errors of design, maintenance, operation, or organization that existed long before the accident occurred. These faults create the background conditions that make possible the evolution of an accident from active error or that amplify the injurious consequences of active error. In other words, latent system failures facilitate the occurrence of active errors, aggravate the extent of injury precipitated by errors, and inhibit normal barriers to iatrogenesis. Wagenaar, Hudson, and Reason have classified system faults into the following general failure types:[14]

- Physical environment (design, missing defenses, hardware defects, negligent maintenance, error-enforcing conditions)
- Human behavior (poor procedures, lack of training)
- Management (incompatible goals, lack of communication)

Work processes, policies, and procedures may be other sources of latent failures.[15] The "safety and quality culture" of an organization can have a notable influence on the care and the attitudes with which personnel perform their tasks.

Latent system faults are present within the system well before the onset of a recognizable accident sequence. The contribution of latent system faults to an accident is usually discovered only after that accident has occurred. Later in this chapter readers are introduced to techniques that can help in identifying and correcting system faults before an accident happens. Such anticipatory failure analysis should be an important component of a hospital's comprehensive patient safety improvement program.

Root Cause Analysis

A root cause analysis begins with outlining the event sequence leading to the accident. Starting with the adverse event itself, the analyst works backward in time, finding and recording each pertinent event. In gathering this information it is important to avoid early judgment, blame, and attribution and to concentrate on the facts of the incident. As each of the actions leading to an event is clearly defined, the investigation team must ask "Why did it occur?" That analysis will contribute to a better understanding of the causal factors in the chain of evolving events.[16] These factors are generally the active precipitating errors.

"How" questions bring the analyst to the root causes or system faults that allowed the active errors to lead to patient injury. During the identification of active errors and latent system faults, the investigation team may be prompted to search for additional information and/or pursue the sequence of events even further back in time.[17] Very often it is not enough to consider only those events that occurred immediately prior to the accident since there may be other causes, more remote in time or in the organization, which must be considered.

The root cause analysis concludes with recommendations for system improvement based on the findings of the investigation. Different methods of root cause analysis vary in emphasis on how the causal factors are decomposed and what changes in the system might be effective in reducing the risk of accidents.

Hospital Accident Investigations

Just as nuclear power plants and airplanes are prone to accidents and disaster when infrastructure subsystems fail, so too are hospitals. Eagle, Davies, and Reason were among the first health care professionals to apply the concepts of active errors and latent system faults in an analysis of a case in which a patient died in an anesthesia mishap.[18] Clinicians erred several times during administration of anesthesia to a 72-year-old man undergoing an elective cystoscopy. First, the initial surgeon determined that the procedure could be done under local anesthesia although the man had a history of confusion and agitation. The patient was switched to general anesthesia when another surgeon assumed care of the patient after admission. However, an adequate preoperative evaluation had not been completed and the anesthesiologist was unaware that the patient had vomited the evening prior to surgery. During the procedure, the patient vomited two liters of gastric contents and aspirated. He died of aspiration pneumonia in six days.

Latent system faults in the hospital's organization of care magnified the ultimate consequences of these human errors. First, double-booking of staff for surgery caused a last-minute change in the surgeon assigned to perform the cystoscopy. Second, the patient's history was maintained in two separate systems—the patient's incident of vomiting the previous night was recorded in a computerized system but not in the medical chart, which was the only source of information available to the surgical team (no computer terminals had been installed in the operating room).

A more recent, larger-scale failure analysis of adverse drug events at two teaching hospitals over a six-month period was reported by Leape and colleagues.[19–21] Sixteen general system faults, in conjunction with human error, contributed to those adverse drug events. Common system faults included deficiencies in drug knowledge dissemination, failure to check drug dose and identity, inadequate or inaccessible information about the patient (such as allergy status) relevant to prescribing, and transcription errors. Many of these failures occurred early in medication management, often at the time that a prescribed medicine was ordered. Thus, injuries to patients resulting from propagation of errors in medication management might be quickly contained by correcting some of these system faults or implementing safety barriers at the drug-ordering step.

Below are analyses of two additional surgical sentinel events.[22] A brief discussion of each case is followed by a listing of what the root cause analysis team identified as active errors and latent system faults.

Case #1

A patient was scheduled for nonurgent surgical repair of an aortic aneurysm. During the early stage of the operation, the surgeon requested that a blood transfusion be started. This was not an urgent or emergent matter; the patient had not experienced significant blood loss. The circulating nurse went to a refrigerator in the operating room and removed a unit of blood from among several units stored there. She looked at the unit label, presumably noting the patient name, and then signed the attestation slip indicating that she recognized the unit as the one prepared for her patient. She handed the blood unit to the anesthesiologist, who immediately started the transfusion without signing the identity affirmation slip. A nurse from an adjoining operating room came to the same refrigerator seeking the blood unit prepared for her patient in the adjourning room who was undergoing a prostatectomy. She noted that the unit was not in the refrigerator and found that the unit she was seeking was, in fact, the one being infused into the patient undergoing the aortic aneurysm repair. The incorrect transfusion was discovered and stopped after only 40 to 50 cc was infused. The patient who received the wrong unit of blood developed coagulopathy and intractable bleeding and later expired.

Active Errors   The death of this patient was precipitated by several active errors. The operating room nurse mistakenly identified the unit of blood selected from the operating room refrigerator as the unit intended for the patient undergoing repair of an aortic aneurysm. The anesthesiologist made a mistake in assuming that the correct unit of blood had been selected and violated safe practices by failing to sign an attestation regarding the accuracy of the blood selection.

Latent System Fault   The organizational policy that allowed storage of the blood for different patients in the same operating room refrigerator created the potential for a catastrophic event. This was a general design fault in the hospital's blood distribution system. This blood storage practice was previously considered safe because it was assumed that several independent persons checking the accuracy of blood selections as well as personally attesting to the accuracy would be an adequate defense against a transfusion administration error.

Case #2

A patient was scheduled for elective surgery for arthroscopic repair of a torn meniscus of the right knee. The hospital leased a CO_2 gas insufflator for distention of the knee joint and an accompanying CO_2 laser beam instrument for use during the procedure. The leasing company provided a technician to assist in the operation of this equipment during surgery. The safety valve on the gas insufflator had been set to release at a low pressure of 2.2 psi. During the surgery there was some difficulty in obtaining adequate gas flow from the insufflator and the technician inadvertently occluded the pressure release valve. For some unknown reason, the company had recently redesigned the equipment and placed the pressure release value in an easily accessible location. The full force of the insufflator, capable of inflating a heavy truck tire, caused CO_2 under pressure to massively dissect upwards from the patient's knee joint, past the tourniquet, and through the peritoneal cavity and diaphragm to the chest. The patient's heart and lungs were compressed; cardiopulmonary failure ensued. After resuscitation and rapid thoracotomy, the patient survived but had severe permanent brain damage.

Active Errors The injury to this patient was precipitated by several active errors in the operation of the gas insufflator. The most egregious error was the unsafe act of the technician when he occluded the insufflator's safety barrier (pressure release value). It was also a mistake for the equipment company to have moved the pressure release valve to a location that made it more likely that tampering could occur.

Latent System Faults Several latent system faults made use of this insufflator an accident waiting to happen. First, the basic design of the insufflator was dubious because it was capable of delivering pressure far exceeding any requirement for its intended use in surgery. Second, the hospital had no procedure for reviewing the design or safe operation of leased equipment prior to its use. Third, training of the technician responsible for operating the insufflator was inadequate and resulted in the penultimate unsafe act.

Summaries of the root cause investigation findings from these two cases are illustrated in figures 4-1 and 4-2.

The occurrence of a sentinel event—an error-initiated accident considered to be particularly egregious in the intensity of its damage to a patient—is a signal that there may be a fault in the organizational policies and procedures that contribute to the event or a deficiency in protective safety procedures that might have prevented the event. The root cause(s) of these common "medical accidents" can be isolated by the methods of analysis that are applied to investigation of accidents in other industries. Once the system faults are identified, corrective action can be taken to reduce the likelihood of future sentinel events.

ANTICIPATORY FAILURE ANALYSIS

Latent system faults can be identified and corrected before a significant injurious patient incident occurs. Evaluating processes within the

Figure 4-1. Root Cause Analysis Results of the Death of a Patient Following Blood Transfusion (Case #1)

Event Sequence	Active Error	Latent System Fault
10. Patient dies		
9. Coagulopathy and hemorrhage		
8. Remedial intervention		
7. Transfusion stopped		
6. Error in transfusion recognized		
5. Blood transfused		
4. Anesthesiologist fails to attest to blood selection	Rule violation	
3. Anesthesiologist assumes blood for the patient has been selected	Mistake	Policy to store blood of different patients in same terminal operating room (OR) refrigerator on day of surgery
2. OR nurse selects blood from terminal OR refrigerator	Mistake	
1. Blood for patient moved from central blood bank to terminal OR refrigerator		

Figure 4-2. Retrospective Root Cause Analysis of Serious Disability Following Elective Arthroscopic Knee Surgery (Case #2)

Event Sequence	Active Error	Latent System Fault
8. Patient suffers serious brain damage		
7. Cardiopulmonary arrest		
6. CO_2 explodes into abdomen and chest		
5. Technician occludes safety valve on insufflator ← Unsafe act ← Absence of training in safe use of equipment		
4. Insufflator inserted into knee, enabled, and restricted flow experienced		
3. Patient received in OR, anesthesia administered		Inadequate policies to ensure safe design and operation of equipment acquired or leased
2. Hospital leases insufflator		
1. Leasing company modifies location of safety valve ← Mistake		

organization to identify where and how an accident might happen is a common activity within private industry. It is as important to conduct similar evaluation within a hospital because of the comparable highly complex nature of patient care activities. As pointed out by Dr. Sven Ternov in chapter 3 of this book, active errors are inevitable. Ongoing "what if" evaluation can highlight recognition of potential accident sequences.

A number of formal anticipatory failure analysis protocols are already in use in private industry. These protocols are generally adapted to particular industrial environments and all analyze to a greater or lesser degree the four elements that characterize hazard systems: source (of hazard), receptors, transmission path, and defensive barriers.[23] Listed below are some of the more common methods:

- Hazop (Hazard and Operability Study) is a hazard-seeking method popular in the chemical process industries.[24] Hazop teams review the design and operation of a facility and identify potential hazards and/or problems with plant operability.
- FMEA (Failure Mode and Effect Analysis) is particularly useful in the prevention of equipment failures.[25] This review starts with a diagram of the operation and includes all components that could possibly fail and conceivably affect the safety of the operation.
- HACCP (Hazard Analysis and Critical Control Point) is a process that is used to monitor food safety.[26] It is a formal method of investigation requiring managerial support and effective training. After defining a process through all stages, every potential hazard is considered (no matter how unlikely), its risk probability evaluated, critical points identified, and effective control monitoring established.
- FTA (Fault Tree Analysis) is a failure analysis method suited to anticipatory study of potential hazards.[27] When used in hazard recognition studies, FTA starts by hypothesizing a specific undesired event, which is graphically placed at the top of an inverted tree diagram. Branches containing potential precursors or causal events (that could lead to the top event) are drawn, extending downward from the top. Additional branching and subbranching are continued down to several levels so as to reach basic causes or primal events for which failure probabilities or failure rates are either available or can be estimated from engineering judgment.

Upon completion of the tree diagram, quantitative evaluation is carried out using the basic primal event failure probabilities or failure rates. FTA is also a particularly useful method of analysis for postaccident investigations.

In chapter 3 of this book, Dr. Sven Ternov briefly discusses Disturbance-Effect-Barrier analysis, an anticipatory failure analysis method that is currently being tested in health care organizations in Sweden. While all of these methods vary somewhat in scope and application, most anticipatory failure analysis activities share several common steps:

- Develop a model of the steps in the process that are potentially subject to failure.
- Ascertain what errors might occur at each step in the process. This requires "what if?" thinking or imaginative simulation of possible disasters.
- Evaluate the hazard potential of errors at each step.
- Isolate any latent system faults that might increase the hazard potential at each step.
- Decide what actions need to take place to lower the hazard potential at each step.

Just as airlines do not want to become famous for the highly efficient way in which they rescue the victims of their crashes, hospitals do not wish to be known for how well they respond to medical accidents.[28] Hospitals cannot afford the loss of reputation or the costs of litigation that arise from adverse event injury to patients. Proactive error reduction efforts are important. Accident prevention, not recovery from accident, is the hallmark of a well-run industry. Every hospital's quality improvement initiative should include anticipatory failure analysis activities.

HOSPITAL PATIENT SAFETY IMPROVEMENT STRUCTURE

Sentinel event occurrence requires root cause analysis. This investigation includes the development of an outline of the details of the event, the description of active failures and possible system and subsystem faults that contributed to the event, identification of actions needed to reduce the risk of another event, and initiation of risk reduction and supporting measurement strategies.

A separate hazard control group is critical to successful implementation of a patient safety program. Each hospital should form a dedicated hazard control group that is given the freedom and accountability to inquire into the safety of hospital operations, analyze sentinel events, and conduct anticipatory failure analysis. The group should consist of people who are knowledgeable about hospital operations and should include a physician, a high-level representative of hospital administration, and a risk manager or quality improvement coordinator. All of them should be trained in the concepts and methods of hazard recognition and accident analysis. Management should be prepared to commit resources to ameliorating system faults identified by this group.

The group would be primarily responsible for evaluating particularly significant, generally infrequent, injury events and near-miss situations. The group should also be charged with conducting prospective failure analyses of circumstances with potential for major injury (sometimes termed *high-risk processes*). Readers will find two chapters in this book (chapters 7 and 8) that describe techniques for measuring and improving high-risk processes. The latent system faults identified by the group should be reported to the medical staff executive committee and hospital administration for review and correction. The hazard control group should also actively promote an organizational culture of hazard recognition, reporting, and correction.

CONCLUSION

Hospital caregivers will commit errors in the course of patient care delivery. These slips, mistakes, and unsafe practices are not intended to cause injury and are often responses to the immediate circumstances involving patient care. "Physicians must make decisions about phenomenally complex problems, under very difficult circumstances, with very little support. They are in the impossible position of not knowing the outcomes of different actions, but having to act anyway."[29] Traditional quality improvement methods have in the past focused on clinician error as a principal causal factor contributing to patient injury. Patient injuries not attributed to clinician error were often dismissed as random, seldom occurring situations.

Hospitals are now turning to the accident investigation methods that have been used by private industry for years. By using root cause analysis techniques, clinicians are learning that error-induced patient injuries often evolve from underlying hospital system faults. By isolating these root causes and correcting them, the risk of future incidents may be diminished. Root cause analysis of sentinel events provides hospital and staff management with information that can be used to make processes more reliable and safe for future patients.

Retrospective root cause analysis, hazard identification, and anticipatory failure analysis require a supportive culture. The commitment of senior management and a willingness to pledge resources are essential. Both management and staff should be familiar with general industry experience that identification and correction of hazards will prevent accidents, minimize injuries, and avert costs attendant to accidents and injuries (lost productivity and litigation). Hospitals must adopt a culture of safety and reliability that places value on procedures, policies, and reward systems that promote error intolerance.

References

1. D. H. Mills et al. *Report on the California Medical Insurance Feasibility Study* (San Francisco, CA: Sutter Publications, 1977).

2. T. A. Brennan et al. "Incidence of Adverse Events and Negligence in Hospitalized Patients: Results of the Harvard Medical Practice Study," *New Engl J Med* 324, no. 6 (1991): 370–76.

3. S. E. Feldman and T. G. Rundall. "PROs and the Health Care Quality Improvement Initiative: Insights From 50 Cases of Serious Medical Mistakes," *Medical Care Review* 50, no. 2 (1993): 123–52.

4. V. C. Marshall and S. Ruhemann. "Anatomy of Hazard Systems and Its Application to Acute Process Hazards," *Trans Instit Chem Engineers* 75, part B (May 1997): 65.

5. P. Spath. "Manage Sentinel Events by Fixing Root Causes," *Hospital Peer Review* 22, no. 12 (1997): 184–88.

6. G. I. Rochlin, T. R. LaPorte, and K. H. Roberts. "The Self-Designing High-Reliability Organization: Aircraft Carrier Flight Operations at Sea," *Naval War College Review* 40, no. 4 (1987): 76–90.

7. K. H. Roberts, ed. *New Challenges to Understanding Organizations* (New York: Macmillan Press, 1993).

8. C. Perrow. *Normal Accidents: Living With High Risk Technologies* (New York: Basic Books, 1984).

9. J. T. Reason. "The Contribution of Latent Human Failures in the Breakdown of Complex Systems," *Philos Trans R Soc Lond* 327B (1990): 475–84.

10. J. T. Reason. *Human Error: Causes and Consequences* (New York: Cambridge University Press, 1990).

11. D. Doerner. "The Logic of Failure," *Philos Trans R Soc Lond* 327B (1990): 463–73.

12. C. Perrow. *Normal Accidents: Living with High Risk Technologies* (New York: Basic Books, 1984).

13. W. A. Wagenaar et al. "Promoting Safety in the Oil Industry," *Ergonomics* 37, no. 12 (1994): 1999–2013.

14. W. A. Wagenaar, P. T. W. Hudson, and J. T. Reason. "Cognitive Failures and Accidents," *Applied Cognitive Psychology* 4, no. 4 (1990): 273–94.

15. R. W. Tuli, G. E. Apostolakis, and J. S. Wu. "Identifying Organizational Deficiencies Through Root-Cause Analysis," *Nuclear Technology* 116, no. 3 (1996): 334.

16. B. S. Lement and J. J. Ferrera. "Accident Causation Analysis by Technical Experts," *J Prod Liability* 5, no. 2 (1982): 145–60.

17. M. Trung Ho. "Accident Analysis and Information System Failure Analysis" in J. A. Wise and A. Debons, eds., *Information Systems Failure Analysis*, NATO ASA Series F32 (Berlin: Springer Verlag, 1987), p. 74.

18. C. J. Eagle, J. M. Davies, and J. T. Reason. "Accident Analysis of Large-Scale Technological Disasters Applied to an Anesthetic Complication," *Can J Anesth* 39, no. 2 (1992): 118–22.

19. L. L. Leape, "Error in Medicine," *JAMA* 272, no. 23 (1994): 1851–57.

20. L. L. Leape et al. "Systems Analysis of Adverse Drug Events," *JAMA* 274, no. 1 (1995): 35–43.

21. D. W. Bates et al. "Incidence of Adverse Drug Events and Potential Adverse Drug Events," *JAMA* 274, no. 1 (1995): 29–34.

22. S. E. Feldman and D. W. Roblin. "Medical Accidents in Hospital Care: Applications of Failure Analysis to Hospital Quality Appraisal," *Jt Comm J on Quality Improvement* 23, no. 11 (November 1997): 567–80.

23. V. C. Marshall and S. Ruhemann. "Anatomy of Hazard Systems and Its Application to Acute Process Hazards," *Trans Instit Chem Engineers* 75, no. 5 (May 1997): 65–72.

24. R. K. Goyal. "Hazops in Industry," *Professional Safety* 38, no. 8 (August 1993): 34–37.

25. G. Kirwan. *A Guide to Practical Human Reliability* (London, Eng.: Taylor & Francis, 1994).

26. G. Palmer. "Hazard Analysis Control Moves into Healthcare," *Manufacturing Chemist* 68, no. 5 (May 1997): 26–27.

27. D. J. Bueker et al. "Fault Tree Analysis of an HCN Pumping System," *Trans Chem* 71, no. 11 (November 1993): 259–68.

28. W. A. Wagenaar. "Profiling Crisis Management," *Journal of Contingencies and Crisis Management* 4, no. 3 (1996): 169–74.

29. D. M. Eddy. "The Challenge," *JAMA* 263, no. 2 (1990): 287–90.

5

Automating Root Cause Analysis

Robert J. Latino

R oot cause analysis (RCA) is a systematic investigation technique that uses information gathered during an intense assessment of an accident to determine the underlying reasons for the deficiencies or failures that caused the accident. RCA techniques have been used for many years in private industry, with the health care industry recently being encouraged by the Joint Commission on Accreditation of Healthcare Organizations to conduct systematic accident investigations.[1] In an industry where human error can mean the difference between life and death, it is essential that health care professionals acquire a clear understanding of the factors that led to an undesirable patient care incident.

Part of developing this understanding involves the use of a disciplined approach such as RCA to study sentinel events, coupled with a means to effectively communicate the results for learning by others. Other chapters in this book describe the process of RCA as it applies to medical accident investigations. The purpose of this chapter is to discuss the benefits of automating this process and what attributes should be considered when evaluating available software packages. Safety experts in private industry have discovered that RCA automation can improve the consistency of accident investigations and help to ensure that appropriate actions are taken to prevent recurrence of similar incidents. Health care providers are likely to find the same benefits.

ADVANTAGES OF RCA AUTOMATION

In an era when computers dominate our lives in every conceivable manner, automating organizationally intensive tasks such as root cause analysis is prudent, effective, and efficient. When we think back before the age of computers about how we used typewriters, for instance, it's hard not to ask ourselves, How did we ever get any work done? We used white-out to hide typographical errors or retyped entire documents to eliminate spelling and grammatical mistakes. Think about how far we've come in such a short time. By using RCA automation technologies, we are taking advantage of a tool that will improve the quality of the analyses and their results while also drastically reducing the time it takes to conduct the investigation.

All of the RCA methods and techniques described in this book outline various means to attain a common end—accurately determining the root causes of a sentinel event. No matter what technique is employed to analyze an event, the underlying theory of cause and effect relationships will always apply. All sentinel events are the result of a series of human errors that queue up in a particular sequence. All of the various automation products available on the market are merely different graphical representations that depict the perceived chain of errors that lead to the undesired outcome. Knowing this, it becomes the analyst's responsibility to evaluate the various automation tools available to determine the best choice for his or her facility. Summarized below are the typical benefits an organization can gain from RCA automation.

Improved Data Organization

Prior to even beginning the evaluation of a sentinel event, analysts should be acutely aware of the objective of doing the investigation and what preparation is necessary to achieve that objective. Preparation usually involves a certain degree of data collection and dissemination. A sentinel event investigator can be likened to a police detective. Why do detectives go to the extent that they do to collect evidence and leads? Many answer that it is to accurately solve the crime. While this is true, we must ask, What is the objective of solving the crime: merely identifying the suspect or obtaining a conviction of the suspect? The only reason that detectives go to the extremes that they do to collect data is because they know they are going to court. And when the case is presented to a lawyer, that lawyer must determine how to present a solid case to the judge and/or jury in order to obtain a conviction. When the evidence collected by the detective is disorganized, the objective— a conviction—is harder to obtain. Organization of data is imperative in any analysis, whether a medical accident investigation or a crime investigation. By automating the data collection process, the root cause analysis team can receive an orderly summary of the preparatory material rather than reams of paper that may be difficult to assimilate.

Reduced Analysis Time

Some RCA methods appear to be cumbersome or too complicated, which may cause the investigation team to lose interest in the process. The sentinel event analysis may drag on with no end in sight. Eventually the analysis is either never completed or completed with unsubstantiated outcomes. Using software to manage an RCA drastically reduces the time necessary for completing it. As an RCA field practitioner myself, I have found that automation generally reduces the accident investigation cycle time by 50 percent.

Improved Rigor

Each organization should have a defined structure for the RCA process, and this structure must be communicated to each RCA team. The problem arises when each team conducts its analysis in a slightly different manner, making it difficult to communicate processes and investigation results with others in the organization. Adherence to a rigorous approach is the bedrock of a worthwhile sentinel event investigation. By standardizing the RCA process, it is easier to make a solid case based on facts. Automation allows the organization to build discipline into the RCA process through the use of established rules that guide the RCA teams through the steps in a consistent manner. Such consistency is likely to improve the accuracy of the team's root cause conclusions.

Easier Reporting Capabilities

In today's health care environment, staff resources are stretched to the limit. While people may find the time to participate on RCA teams, when the work of the team is done, someone must take time to develop the final sentinel event investigation report. The report of the team's findings is one of the most crucial elements of the entire RCA process. Not only does the report substantiate the need for internal changes, it also helps in meeting the accreditation standards of the Joint Commission. If the entire RCA process is automated, the report can be automatically generated immediately following the end of the investigation.

Enhanced Follow-up Capabilities

The final advantage of automating the RCA process is to improve the follow-up process. With every sentinel event investigation, something is expected to improve as a result of the effort. Once the action plans are implemented, the effectiveness of the actions must be measured. By automating the follow-up process, data can be easily entered into the software program to quickly illustrate where improvements have occurred or where additional work is needed.

DESIRABLE FEATURES

The features to look for in an RCA software program will vary somewhat depending on the model chosen. Because the Joint Commission has not currently mandated one specific prototype for conducting an RCA, each facility may have a slightly different process for conducting the investigation. While many RCA methods exist, most demonstrate similar key steps. Discussed below are the general factors that companies in private industry tend to look for when purchasing RCA software packages. Many of these same features are likely to be important to health care organizations, regardless of the RCA model they've chosen to adopt.

Reactive versus Proactive Analysis

The selection of the proper analytical tool to use depends greatly on the focus of the analysis. Will the software program be used to support the investigation of an event that has already occurred (such as a sentinel event), or will it be used proactively to minimize the risk of a potential occurrence? Traditionally, RCA has been applied to the investigation of historical occurrences, whereas methods such as Failure Modes, Effects, and Criticality Analysis (FMECA) deal with probabilistic occurrences.[2]

Reactive and proactive safety management strategies, however, are complementary, not contradictory. A good overall strategy should involve the goal of eliminating undesirable outcomes, not merely responding to events after the fact. Risk assessment tools help minimize the likelihood of undesirable outcomes, whereas RCA strives to eliminate the recurrence of past undesirable events.

Some automated accident investigation techniques can be used under both circumstances with a knowledgeable analyst facilitating the process. Keep in mind that no matter which technique is used, these software tools are about 95 percent dependent on how the user interprets the risk reduction process.

Simplistic

There is a common paradigm seen in any industry whereby people believe that because the problem seems extremely complex, then an equally complex approach for solving it is necessary. This paradigm does not apply to RCA software. Look for the software product that is the simplest to follow and is not overloaded with features and capabilities that will rarely be used. Think about how many features of Microsoft™ Word the majority of users actually use compared with the many features available. Probably very few of the features are routinely used. Apply the same principle in your search for RCA software. First, determine what your needs are for conducting the analysis. Next, convert those needs into automation features that are necessary for meeting your needs. Then evaluate the available software products based on your selected features.

Objective

The identification of root causes following a sentinel event can be a very subjective activity. This subjectivity can introduce human error into the analysis process itself. The RCA team members must remain unbiased and separate facts from assumptions. Because of the subjectivity of evaluating hypotheses developed during an RCA, seek out some intuitive features in the software.

All software programming involves the development of rules, which allow or prevent users to perform or not perform certain tasks. RCA software is no different. The selected software should guide the RCA team through such processes as selecting causes and determining effect. Another important rule is that all hypotheses (possible causes) must be proven or disproved with factual data rather than relying on hearsay alone. Search for the RCA software that systematically guides the RCA team through the investigation process; otherwise the team may guide the project to where the team would like it to end up rather than to its logical conclusion.

Comprehensive

If you have ever had to perform RCAs manually, you will surely appreciate the value of automation when its comes to comprehensiveness. Typically, a manual RCA may involve several different software programs. For example, the text portion of the report might be written on a word processing program; a flowcharting program might be used to illustrate the sequence of the events leading up to the accident; presentation software might be used to create the RCA report for the quality council. One RCA software package should include integrated capabilities for all of these functions.

Most automated RCA methods have the same basic elements: data collection and organization, team member selection, logic sequence representation, validation of hypotheses, identification of causes, and recommendations. You may want the software to include such features as a standardized report writer, presentation development capabilities, and ability to track improvements based on implemented recommendations. Such features help the quality or risk manager perform the needed oversight functions.

Organized

The software should support the RCA method selected by the organization. This feature makes the software attractive to the administrators who oversee the RCA team because they can easily follow the flow of the investigation and can quickly review the RCA electronic file for updates on the team's progress.

Flexible

RCAs have been formally performed in industrial settings for decades. These accident investigations have been primarily prompted by regulations enforced by the Occupational Safety and Health Agency (OSHA), the Environmental Protection Agency (EPA), and a host of other groups. Most RCA software on the market today uses industrial language/terminology. The software selected should be easily translatable into the health care field. Some vendors are customizing their products to meet the needs of the health care industry.

Adequate Reporting Capabilities

The organization must determine what will be required of them in terms of reporting RCA findings and who will review these reports. The selected RCA software should be able to support organizational needs and provide both detailed and high-level reporting. Ideally, it should not be necessary to export information from the RCA software program into another program (such as a spreadsheet or word processing program) in order to create reports.

RCA Training

Most RCA software programs have been developed by RCA consulting firms who also provide training in how to use the software for field applications. Determine if employees will need training in RCA and whether the selected software vendor provides such training. Chances are that the firms that provide specific RCA software are companies that will support it in the field and be available for consulting on RCA issues.

Value

The cost of the software package is one thing, value is another! The organization must first determine its needs and then determine which software package best suits these needs. At this point, cost of the product is considered. Value is determined when the anticipated returns of using the selected products are weighed against the initial purchase price. Anticipated returns can be intrinsic (for example, less time needed to conduct the RCA and improved data collection and organization steps) or extrinsic (for example, quick, accurate conclusions will reduce/eliminate the risk of incident recurrence). Value is in the eyes of the user. Evaluating software strictly on cost alone could cause you to overlook the most suitable product for your needs.

RCA SOFTWARE CHOICES

There are several software products that support basic graphics and flowcharting functions. Although they are not specifically designed for RCA, they can be used to automate one or more steps of the accident investigation. There are also numerous vendors of environmental, health, and safety applications. These software applications are geared toward compliance with regulatory statutes imposed by agencies such as the Nuclear Regulatory Commission, EPA, OSHA, Department of Energy, Department of Defense, and others. These products primarily automate the internal risk assessment process and are not intended to be used for retrospective RCA of actual occurrences.

The companies listed below have designed software that automate the steps of a formal root cause analysis that would be conducted following a significant adverse event. These products have been used for several years in private industry.

Decision Systems, Inc.
802 N. High St., Suite C
Longview, TX 75601
(903) 236-9973; Web site: http://www.rootcause.com
RCA software: REASON

JBF Associates, Inc.
1000 Technology Dr.
Knoxville, TN 37932
(423) 966-5232; Web site: http://www.jbfa.com
RCA software: BRAVO

Reliability Center, Inc.
P.O. Box 1421
Hopewell, VA 23860
(804) 458-0645; Web site: http://www.reliability.com
RCA software: PROACT

System Improvements, Inc.
238 S. Peters Rd., Suite 301
Knoxville, TN 37923-5224
(615) 539-2139; Web site: http://www.taproot.com
RCA software: TAPROOT

Organizations seeking RCA automation alternatives are encouraged
to contact all of the above software vendors to obtain a demonstration
version of their product. Then use the list of desirable attributes found
earlier in this chapter to determine the best choice for your current
circumstances.

No matter what RCA software is chosen, it is up to the user to make
it work. Automation tools are developed to make performing the task
easier for the user; automation of the task does not replace the need for
people to think. The software product supplies the RCA team with a
means to logically deduce a series of occurrences or a sequence of
errors. Although the methods and tools will help formulate and structure the thought process, humans are still required to input factual data
and observations. Like any automated system, if the input is nonsense,
the output will be no better.

CONCLUSION

Each organization should define its own method for conducting a root
cause analysis following an accident. If a formal method has not been
agreed on, accident investigations are likely to yield inconsistent results
and miscommunications because of the lack of consistency. If not for-
malized, people will develop their own systems for organizing, documenting, and reporting RCA results. In my experience, many accident
investigations fail to achieve the desired outcomes because people cannot effectively communicate. Without structure, the RCA process
becomes sporadic, inconclusive, and subjective.

Automation brings consistency to the table, resulting in standardization of the RCA process, documentation, presentation, and results. Automation increases individual productivity because it expedites the cycle time necessary for conducting an RCA. Having an automated system also allows the analyst to demonstrate progress at any point during the investigation. The use of electronic files allows data to be transferred to other team members, decision makers, regulatory authorities, or whoever else the analyst feels should have the information.

Many health care systems, such as the Veterans Health Administration, are working to develop a database of root cause analysis findings from their member facilities.[3] This is an admirable goal as individual facilities will be able to learn from the experiences of others. The Joint Commission is attempting to create such a database on a nationwide scale.[4] The overall goal of conducting any RCA should be to prevent recurrence of the event in any facility, not just the one in which the incident occurred. This means that the new knowledge gained from one organization's root cause analysis should be shared with other facilities. However, the development of such a database will be difficult if the reporting formats are not consistent and nearly impossible if the information is not automated. With the many new computing technologies, organizations now have the ability to share information with specific parties around the world in a matter of seconds. If the goal of shared learning is to be realized, RCA automation at the facility level is essential.

References

1. "Policy for Evaluating Occurrence of 'Sentinel Events' Established," *Joint Commission Perspectives* 16, no. 1 (1996): 6.

2. Ronald T. Anderson and Lewis Neri. *Reliability-Centered Maintenance* (New York: Elsevier Science Publishers, Ltd., 1990), pp. 132–35.

3. Statement of Thomas L. Garthwaite, MD, Deputy Under Secretary for Health Department of Veterans Affairs on VA's Risk Management Program before the Subcommittee on Oversight & Investigations Committee on Veterans' Affairs, U.S. House of Representatives (May 14, 1998).

4. "Special Report on Sentinel Events," *Joint Commission Perspectives* 18, no. 6 (November/December 1998): 19–38.

6

One Hospital's View of Software Facilitation of Root Cause Analysis

Kenneth A. Hirsch, MD, PhD

Dennis T. Wallace, DABRM

When the Joint Commission on Accreditation of Healthcare Organizations expanded its requirements to include root cause analyses of sentinel events, our facility, a major medical center in southern California, began to include this process in its continuous quality improvement efforts. Although root cause analysis is new to health care systems, it is well respected and accepted in a variety of industrial risk management arenas. As addressed in more detail elsewhere in this book, root cause analysis is a set of steps by which the underlying causes of adverse outcomes may be identified with the goal of preventing the recurrence of such events. The Joint Commission has been explicit in defining the situations that are considered reviewable by their organization. These are any events that result in a serious patient injury or death.[1] Like most facilities, our medical center has chosen to conduct root cause analyses on selected near-miss situations in addition to those events considered reviewable by the Joint Commission. As of June 1999, root cause analyses had been conducted on 11 patient incidents within the mental health service line, with only one being a sentinel event by Joint Commission criteria.

Because root cause analyses were expanding the scope and function of traditional continuous quality improvement activities, it became necessary for the medical center to identify a process that was both efficient and effective. It was during the development of this process that the organization explored root cause analysis (RCA) computerization options. The purpose of this chapter is to describe the factors that the physicians and staff at our medical center believe are important to consider in evaluating RCA software packages for use in the health care setting. The results of our preliminary analysis of current RCA software products will also be presented. It is important to point out that the automation features that we felt to be crucial may not be as important to other health care facilities. The purchase decisions of an organization should be based on the specific, identified, and prioritized needs of the end users.

VALUE OF AUTOMATION

After completing our first RCA "manually," we sought out a software product that would facilitate and enhance the effectiveness and efficiency of the process. We found the Joint Commission's manual, *How to Conduct a Root Cause Analysis in Response to a Sentinel Event*, to be a useful starting point in learning about the RCA analytic process. However, we encountered enormous difficulty when we tried to translate this model into an efficacious, efficient, and cost-effective standardized procedure. This challenge was compounded by the variety of analytic tools that may be used during the performance of root cause analyses. We hoped to find the ideal software product that would guide an essentially untrained or minimally trained analysis team through each RCA step.

In any endeavor in which there are sequential and iterative steps to be followed, a standardized process by which that activity may be enacted generally is beneficial in terms of validity and cost-effectiveness. Automation of such activities offers the advantages of data storage and manipulation as well as assistance in guiding individuals through the process steps. This same argument can be made for the activity of root cause analysis.

Cost avoidance is an important additional consideration. The medical center estimated that its first root cause analysis (a very simple one) cost approximately $8,000 in direct salary costs. This estimate did not include the indirect costs related to lost clinical service availability, support services, and so on. At the halfway point in another investigation (this time a more serious incident), costs were estimated to be approximately $13,000 in direct salary expenditures and $23,000 in lost revenues. After completing several root cause analyses manually, it rapidly became clear that a standardized process that was easy to follow had to be developed. Otherwise, for cost reasons alone people would perform root cause analyses in a pro forma manner just to satisfy accreditation requirements with minimal impact on patient care.

An adverse event with a poor outcome could easily invite a malpractice lawsuit from an injured and angry patient. A well-done, credible RCA can be very valuable in mitigating loss from professional liability claims. It can also assist in planning for the defense of a malpractice suit against the named practitioner and/or the health care organization responsible for the patient's care and safety. The RCA would greatly assist the defendant's legal team in preparing and presenting its defense. We have observed hospital attorneys encouraging the performance of a root cause analysis in response to an adverse event or outcome. Since automation of an RCA can theoretically produce consistently higher-quality analyses, stronger defensive postures can be formulated that decrease the risk of resource losses.

RCA SOFTWARE EVALUATION CRITERIA

There already exists in private industries an assortment of software packages designed to facilitate all or part of the RCA process. A variety of nomenclature (fault tree, failure mode, and so on) are used, and many different RCA models are available. Products range from those vendors offering a single-focus product (for example, factor and impact weighting in an otherwise completed root cause analysis) to those products that purport to guide users through an entire RCA from problem statement to solution impact assessment. Given the very limited level of sophistication of RCA techniques in the health care industry and the urgency with which that industry is being "encouraged" or, indeed, mandated to embrace this continuous improvement tool, it is the more comprehensive software products that are likely to be most desirable.

It was believed at the medical center that the use of software to facilitate the RCA process would offer advantages in a number of realms. If the steps of the RCA could be standardized, greater efficiency would result. Although standardization does not require automation (a detailed procedure with explicit instructions would ensure a consistent analytic procedure), a well-designed software program could eliminate the need to develop such an internal procedure and similarly eliminate the need to define a process with which we were relative novices. Data organization and collection would be simplified if the software program were to include, for example, a relational database structure that allowed for data collection, analysis, and review. Report generation would also be simplified. Ideally, an RCA software product would guide us in the development of output that could meet all internal and external reporting needs without violating the integrity of the data or the analytic process. In essence, we hoped to find an RCA software product that would decrease learning time; shorten the analytic process; increase validity of the process by providing an external expertise and instilling procedural consistency; facilitate collection, analysis, and presentation of data; increase the depth of study; and guide the production of meaningful reports, including post-RCA monitoring.

We started our search for the ideal RCA software product by identifying a series of requirements unique to our facility for the product we hoped to acquire. The requirements evolved as we became more knowledgeable about root cause analysis. The latest set of requirements for the medical center are listed below. The reader is cautioned, however, that the necessary software features will vary according to the specific needs of any given facility or group of users. Our criteria are presented as a starting point for discussions in other organizations and are not intended to establish an industry standard.

Philosophy

Given the resistance that may be encountered regarding the performance of root cause analyses in any form, it was considered critical that the software in no way increase that resistance. In practical terms, this means that there should be nothing in the program flow that conflicts with what we viewed as important error-reduction philosophies in health care, which include the following:

- There should be no presumption of human error evident in the program's logic structure.

- Contributing factors as well as causative factors should be sought for each event.
- Contributing or partial solutions should be allowed, even welcomed.

Windows Compliant

It was believed unreasonable to expect that an RCA program would also possess fully featured word processor and presentation capabilities. Windows compliance with full support for drag-and-drop interface was felt to be necessary to eliminate the need to retype content into other software programs. Given operating system development and migration expectations, the software would have to operate under Windows 95a, 95b, 98, and NT. For ease and flexibility of use, full OLE (object linking and embedding) capability, standard Windows controls, and other similar features were believed to be necessary.

Ease of Use

Another factor facilitating ease of use besides Windows compliance would involve the overall structure of the program and the logic of the data flow. These had to be intuitive. The typical user would be an infrequent participant in RCA and would not be able or willing to spend significant time learning basic software functionalities. The typical user would also not wish to read a training manual (a behavior observed in users of most new software developed today) and therefore we wanted the RCA software to include a quick-start guide or its equivalent, supported by on-line help as well as a user's manual. Because few hospital personnel would be working with the RCA software on a regular basis, the software's intuitive ease of use was felt to be critical.

Data Entry

Another factor in ease of use is the requirement that a data element should require entering only once. As the user progresses from one module to another, data elements should be automatically carried forward, thereby minimizing redundant data entry. In addition, the software should not unduly limit the length of any given data field. It was felt that data fields should allow entries of at least 250 characters even in the graphic module.

Terminology

Despite the fact that the RCA software programs we examined were all designed for industries other than health care, it was critical that the nomenclature be relatively understandable. While it was recognized that some process-specific terminology was unavoidable, the program should allow the user to complete a root cause analysis without having to learn a new language. It was believed that terms from private industry RCA, such as *latent cause*, *failure mode*, and *relative generating causality*, might inhibit caregivers' use of the program and therefore interfere with the effectiveness of the RCA. Similarly, an overabundance of engineering or industrial safety terminology was felt to be disadvantageous (*scram*, *channel capacity*, and so on). Even if the typical health care RCA team member could grasp the meaning of these terms, he or she might be dissuaded from using the software. We hoped to find an RCA software program that would allow our facility to modify the terminology appearing on screens, buttons, and so on in order to match the RCA terms used in our facility.

Validity

The RCA software program would in some way have to help protect novice users from drawing incomplete or inaccurate conclusions. In essence, the software should walk the analysis team through the RCA process from start to finish with protective queries and safeguards along the way. This should start with problem or event identification and team composition and continue through final reporting. This concern was highlighted in our examination of one RCA software product that appeared initially to be a viable product for our use. On further examination, it became evident that while giving the impression of having led the user to a valid set of conclusions, the RCA was in fact not felt to be credible and thorough. People inexperienced in the RCA process could easily end up with an incomplete analysis while all the time believing in the validity of the findings. It was recognized that this is a very difficult expectation for software developers to meet, especially since even the Joint Commission seems, in our opinion, to be unable to objectively define the difference between a credible and noncredible RCA. Nonetheless, this feature was believed to be among the most important.

Noncontributing Factors

In a true sense, factors that do not contribute to the occurrence of an adverse event have no role in a root cause analysis—they are, in essence, ruled out during the investigation. It is often critical, nonetheless, to document those factors simply to verify that they were explored and found not to be relevant. This finding may be particularly important to document in the reports shared with senior management and litigators. Explaining why specific, common, potential contributing factors do not apply in a given sentinel event situation may also be useful when communicating with regulatory or accreditation groups such as the Joint Commission.[2] The ability to include such factors in the computerized RCA causal factors listing and extract them for reporting purposes is crucial.

Tools

Because the performance of an RCA involves the use of a number of analytic and group consensus tools, the program should guide users through the use of these tools in the appropriate RCA analytic sequence, and the results should become part of the RCA report. At our institution we specifically wanted tools for the following activities: event sequencing, brainstorming and affinitization, barrier identification, and contributory factor diagrams. Other organizations may want the software program to include tools for barrier analysis, change analysis, cause-and-effect diagrams, or other RCA techniques.

Operational Logic Flow

The program should lead the analysis team through each step in the RCA analytic process using the data from prior sections or modules to initiate the next sections in a progressive manner. The software should provide for entry of a full description of the adverse event under investigation. Optimally this would entail a brief narrative entry to begin the process, followed by a detailed sequence of events to be generated by the analysis team as the RCA is conducted. This detailed sequence of events would provide a starting point for the actual investigation. For example, by asking the question why or how for each step in the event chain, the RCA team would be able to identify both causal and contributing factors and then proceed to the selection of root causes. The software should prompt the analysis team for general categories of causal, contributing, and root causes in order to reduce the likelihood of factors being overlooked. Corrective opportunities, implementation plan, and validation of intervention effectiveness should all be addressed in the progressive steps through which the software guides the team.

Training Capacity

Although it was expected that a very limited number of hospital personnel would become formally trained in the performance of RCA, we looked to the software itself to be a training tool. We wanted the program to teach the novice user the process of conducting a RCA, in addition to having the software make life easier for the individual or team that is already expert in the process. We felt so strongly about the training aspects that if a company recommended formal training in the use of its software (as opposed to seminars on root cause analysis in general), we took this as an indication that the product would be too complex for our needs. It would not be sufficiently intuitive and user-friendly.

Output

A variety of reports are needed during an RCA plus at least one comprehensive report at the end of the investigation that can be exported to other Windows-based programs for modification. The final report should include all RCA information from the problem statement to final recommendations. Our medical center uses the FOCUS-PDCA model of continuous improvement and looked for software that could support this reporting format. Ideally, the program would afford the user a menu of reporting choices and formats. A special function report we particularly wanted was one that would show a cost accounting of how much the analysis actually cost the organization, reporting both direct and indirect RCA costs (for example, staff hours expended, salaries, and lost productivity time). Such data would enable senior management to better assess the cost of quality improvement versus the cost of maintaining the status quo.

Graphics

The graphics capabilities of the program should include a "shape library" that allows users to define shape and color coding for various factors and factor categories. This was believed important in order to improve the ease of comprehension of the graphic images (whether a flowchart, a cause-and-effect diagram, events and causal factors chart, or another graphic). Our preference was for a tree structure contributory factor diagram, with the adverse event at the top, root causes at the bottom, and connecting steps in between ("contributing" and "causal" factors).[3] We prefer this graphic tree structure because it is easy for the analyst to quickly evaluate the thoroughness and credibility of the RCA. Root causes are easily identified as are corrective action opportunities. Each level of the tree documents the team's response to "why" questions and the resultant answers. We have experimented with several graphic displays for reporting analyses in the manner described above with very impressive results. Because visual presentation of the RCA is a very potent aid to both comprehension and impact, we feel that a good software package should provide strong graphics functionality to support the contributory factor diagram chart chosen for use by our facility.

Database Functionality

The program should be able to provide two distinct database capabilities. All RCA reports will likely be submitted to, and maintained by, the risk management or quality management offices and specific departments of a given facility. The RCA database structure should provide for access to any entire root cause analysis and separately should also allow access to a collection (database tables) of common elements that may be useful to analysis teams from different departments. Distinct from this, the risk manager or quality management personnel will need a means of tracking the status of all root cause analyses within the facility, with the ability to track RCA projects within specific departments or functional areas. Department-specific RCA status tracking would involve the ability to determine whether the recommendations of a specific RCA analysis had been implemented or follow-up analysis begun. Users should be able to create special reports using these databases.

Search Function

The RCA software program should possess text search capabilities for both analyses currently under way and those already completed.

LAN Capabilities/Data Integration

Increasingly, health care facilities are using more advanced communication and automation technologies, especially local area networks (LANs), including intranets, shared databases, and so on. The software should be capable of operating in a secure mode in a LAN environment. In addition, however, since some facilities and some users would be using the program separate from direct LAN connection (for example, notebook computer at an RCA meeting), the program should allow for such remote operation even on a LAN license and should further provide for integration of data and reports from within the LAN and information imported from stand-alone computers.

Confidentiality

All quality improvement material, including RCA reports, should be maintained in a secure environment without identifiers, especially patient and provider identifiers. The RCA software program should provide a means of coding pertinent identifiers with access to that coding restricted by the program's security functionality. This confidentiality is necessary to protect patients, the facility, and the staff. Without such security, the likelihood of full, open, and voluntary participation in the RCA process diminishes rapidly.

Hierarchical Security

It is important that access to identifying data codes, root cause analyses, the database maintaining the status of those analyses, and the ability to set certain user preferences (selection of terminology on program screens and so forth) be controlled. At least three levels of hierarchical security would be needed to ensure this control.

Cost

RCA software is relatively inexpensive (approximate price range of $600 to $1,200). The prices for RCA programs currently on the market are all far less than the cost of doing a single root cause analysis manually. Therefore, software functionality becomes the primary determinant. Even when one considers the strong likelihood of an average-sized health care organization needing several copies of the selected program (or multiple-user LAN license), the price range appeared to us to be a relatively minor consideration compared to the desired capabilities.

Readers are reminded again that the features listed above represent what our medical center believed to be important in selecting an RCA software product. Other facilities may have different factors on their software want list. Once your organization has listed all desirable RCA software features, people who are familiar with the selection criteria should prioritize each factor according to its criticality. Table 6-1 can be used for this exercise. Listed in the table are the selection criteria felt to be important by our facility. Space is provided to list other criteria. Determine which attributes are crucial (must have), important (want to have), and desirable (nice to have). Use the results of a multivoting process to evaluate the adequacy of various RCA software products. It is unlikely that the entire list of features will be available in one software package. By ranking the importance of each feature, the team can pinpoint the products most likely to contain the facility's principal requirements for an RCA software package.

MATCHING FEATURES WITH PRODUCTS

In mid-1998 our risk management department, together with medical staff representatives, evaluated the software products currently available from

Table 6-1.   Matrix to Use in Setting Priorities for RCA Software Features

Feature	Crucial	Important	Desirable
Error-reduction philosophy consistent with that of facility			
Windows compliant			
Logical flow/on-line help			
Nonduplicative data entry/sufficiently large data fields			
Minimal use of industrial RCA terminology/ customization capabilities			
Safeguards to protect the validity of the RCA process			
Ability to enter and save data about noncontributing factors			
Preferred analytic and group consensus tools			
Logical operational flow			
Able to train novices in the RCA process			
Output includes desired content and in chosen format			
Graphics capabilities that can be customized to facility's needs			
Interrelationship database functionality			
Search capabilities			
Local area network/data integration capabilities			
Ability to protect the confidentiality of patients, providers, and other pertinent RCA details			
Hierarchical security			

several companies. These software packages included PHA-Pro,[4] PROACT,[5] REASON,[6] TapRooT,[7] FaultTree+,[8] CARA-FaultTree,[9] BRAVO,[10] and SAPHIRE.[11] At the time these products were reviewed, none of the vendors had developed a health care version of their software. After extensively testing these RCA software programs we purchased none. No software program appeared to meet even half of the requirements that we felt to be the most crucial. We also compared the output from the software programs with several actual RCAs we had done without the assistance of automation. In terms of the quality of results and efficiency, the nonautomated RCA methodology was felt to be superior and was preferred by our staff.

CONCLUSION

At the time this chapter was prepared (June 1999), the RCAs at our medical center were still being performed manually using performance improvement tools, process facilitators, and a combination of word processors and flowcharting software, plus our own locally developed RCA training manual. We are aware that at least two of the RCA products that we evaluated in mid-1998 are undergoing revision to accommodate the needs of the health care market. In addition, a new RCA software product, Root Cause Analyst, is currently being developed jointly by a medical risk management firm and a company specializing in software for behavioral medicine, with commercial release expected in September 1999.[12] By the time this book is published, this product may be available for purchase.

Because automation can bring many benefits to the RCA process in health care, it is our hope that updated versions of existing products or perhaps totally new products designed specifically for the health care industry will eventually be able to meet our RCA software requirements.

References

1. "Special Report on Sentinel Events," *Joint Commission Perspectives* 18, no. 6 (November/December 1998): 29.

2. P. Spath. *Investigating Sentinel Events: How to Find and Resolve Root Causes* (Forest Grove, OR: Brown-Spath & Associates, 1997), p. 40.

3. M. Ammerman. *The Root Cause Analysis Handbook* (New York: Quality Resources, 1998), pp. 37–41.

4. PHA-Pro is marketed by Dyadem International Ltd., Markham, Ontario; 905-940-1600; Web site: http://www.dyadem.com.

5. PROACT is marketed by Reliability Center, Inc., Hopewell, VA; 804-458-0645; Web site: http://www.reliability.com.

6. REASON is marketed by Decision Systems, Inc., Longview, TX; 903-236-9973; Web site: http://www.rootcause.com.

7. TapRooT is marketed by System Improvements, Inc., Knoxville, TN; 423-539-2139; Web site: http://www.taproot.com.

8. FaultTree+ is marketed by Item Software Corporation, Hampshire, U.K.; Telephone: +44 (0) 1489 885085; Web site: http://www.maintainability.com/safety.html.

9. CARA-FaultTree is marketed by SINTEF Industrial Management, Trondheim, Norway; Telephone: +47 73 59 27 56; Web site: http://www.sintef.no/sipaa/prosjekt/cara/cft.html.

10. BRAVO is marketed by ABS Group Inc., Risk & Reliability Division, Knoxville, TN; 423-671-5813; Web site: http://www.jbfa.com/bravo.html.

11. SAPHIRE information and software is available from sources identified on the SAPHIRE Users Group Web site: http://sageftp.inel.gov/saphire/saphire.asp.

12. The software Root Cause Analyst is being developed by Medical Risk Management Associates, LLC, San Diego, CA, telephone 877-816-6594; and Accurate Assessments, Inc., Omaha, NE; 800-324-7966; Web site: http://www.sentinel-event.com.

7

Proactively Error-Proofing Health Care Processes

Richard J. Croteau, MD

Paul M. Schyve, MD

In health care, the occurrence of a sentinel event is compelling. A response is demanded, driven in some cases by guilt, shame, or fear of retribution; in other instances by a need to understand and correct the problem. That response can be limited to the placement of blame and removal of the offending party. Or through the process of a root cause analysis, people can achieve an understanding of the factors that enabled the event to occur. Such an analysis may lead to process redesign to reduce the risk of that type of event in the future. However, even a root cause analysis, with all its potential for reducing risk, can itself be limited by the "blinder" effect of the specific event. The best root cause analyses look not only at the factors surrounding the specific event, but also at the entire process that was involved and its support systems. The goal of a good root cause analysis should be to minimize overall risk associated with that process, not just recurrence of the event that prompted the investigation. The event itself serves only as a flag: "Risky process here!" It signals an opportunity to reduce overall risk and provides the motivation to do so. Having served that purpose, the event, although potentially useful as a reference point, is no longer necessary to the analysis and redesign of the overall process.

So why wait for a sentinel event before processes are improved? Surely we can identify processes that are high risk through our own and others' experience. The purpose of this chapter is to explore the possibilities for proactively assessing and minimizing risk. These activities are perhaps less compelling than responding to an actual event unless one sees this activity in the context of not a single event but of the overall, unacceptably high frequency of sentinel events in all of health care.

ANATOMY AND PHYSIOLOGY OF A PROCESS

Aspiring clinicians are taught extensively about the human body: what can go wrong with it and what can be done to protect it. They learn these lessons in order to prevent things from going wrong and to treat it when things do go wrong. But these curricula have included little or nothing about what can go wrong with the process of providing that care. Clinicians study the recipients of health care but not the anatomy, normal physiology, pathology, prevention, and treatment of what they personally do as health care professionals.

Let's try to understand what health care professionals do by using a model that clinicians are already familiar with: structure (anatomy), function (physiology), dysfunction (pathology), treatment (health promotion, disease prevention, active treatment, palliation, and rehabilitation), and maintenance (follow-up care) as these concepts apply to health care processes. The analogy may suffer somewhat because of the way we relate to the participants. In studying disease, the immediate participant is the patient. And we have, for the most part, tended not to blame the patient for his or her disease. Health care processes, on the other hand, involve a number of participants whom we still have a tendency to blame when the process breaks down. Perhaps it would be instructive for the moment to suspend the concept of blame in our thoughts about the function or dysfunction of health care processes.

The dictionary definition of a process, "a systematic series of actions directed to some end," provides some insight into the structure, function, and potential risk points of a process that can be useful in formulating an approach to proactive risk reduction.[1] *Systematic* implies regularity or consistency; *series* tells us that there is some order, that the parts are related in some way. *Actions* are things to be done, forcing the question, By whom or what? (This is where we sometimes wander down the path to blame and retribution.) *Directed* suggests intent, design, or plan to achieve *some end* (the desired outcome). The anatomy then is the totality of the parts of the process—the actions or steps—and their sequence. As with the human body or a machine, a part can fail (a bone can break, a tire can blow out) but the effect of the failure is most often determined by how the parts interact, how the function of the process (or body, or machine) is affected. The physiology of a process is how it functions; how the parts work together to produce the desired effect. Each step in the process requires an input—delivered on time, complete, and in usable form—and yields an output—a product of that step in the process. This output is often the input for another step in the process.

HOW PROCESSES FAIL

Given the structure and function of a process, what kind of pathology might we expect to see? Consider a relay race with four runners, each making one lap around the track, each in top physical condition, each a well-trained, experienced runner. What can go wrong? A trip. A cramp. Did I mention the baton? Oh yes, in a relay race, continuity is important. The baton represents the deliverable to be handed off from one runner to the other. The winning team is not necessarily the one with the fastest individual times; it is often the one with the most efficient and reliable hand-offs. It is the interaction between the racers that most often determines the outcome. And an error in transferring the baton is much more likely than a runner tripping or getting a leg cramp!

So what does this mean for our process? Certainly the anatomy can be flawed; that is, a step in the process is poorly designed. If the process is designed from the outset to do something different from the desired result (that is, a primary design flaw that could be considered a congenital defect in the process), the results will be more or less consistently undesirable. But far more often, the failure of a process to achieve its designed objective has to do with the design of the linkages between steps in the process: how the steps relate to one another—the hand-offs. It is the interrelationships that are themselves prone to failure and that propagate the effects of a failure to other parts of the process, often in ways that are unexpected (side effects) or not immediately evident (long-term effects).

There are, of course, factors outside the process itself that can influence the outcome. And while these may not be subject to our direct control, they can nonetheless be identified and their influences on our process understood and protected against. Such an external factor may be a special cause of variation in the process under review and therefore generally cannot be controlled through redesign of the process itself.[2] However, such a special cause may, and often should, lead us to assess and redesign factors external to the process that *are* under our control or to redesign our process to protect it against those factors that are *not* under our control.

Whether any cause is common or special depends on the frame of reference. That is, the concepts of "common" and "special" are not attributes of a cause but rather express the relationship of a specific cause to a specific process. For example, a patient's death may result from the loss of electrical power during a surgical procedure. While this undesirable variation in outcome is the result of a special cause in the operating room, the special cause is, in turn, the result of a common cause in the organization's system for preparing for a utility failure. In fact, often a special cause of variation in one process will be found to be the result of a common cause of variation in the larger system (that is, larger set of processes) of which the immediate process is a part.

This analysis leads to the conclusion that the identification of a special cause for a sentinel event is only the first step in a full evaluation of the event. The second step is to identify the larger system whose common cause variation is the source of the special cause. It is this larger system that then becomes the focus for improvement, because only it can be redesigned to eliminate the common cause of the adverse event. The component process cannot correct a special cause in itself.

Continuation of this analytical process, as depicted in figure 7-1, will eventually lead to factors that are outside the control of the organization itself. These external environmental factors—whether physical, social, economic, political, or other—may correctly be identified as the ultimate root causes. However, these factors are largely beyond the control of the individual organization. The organization's corrective actions should again focus on its own internal systems because only they can be redesigned to reduce risk; in this case by acknowledging the realities of uncontrollable external environmental factors, anticipating their impact on the organization, and redesigning to protect against the effects of those external factors.

What does this mean for health care organizations? All clinical processes in the organization are part of larger systems in the organization. Thus, special cause sentinel events that occur in the care of

Figure 7-1.   Levels of Analysis

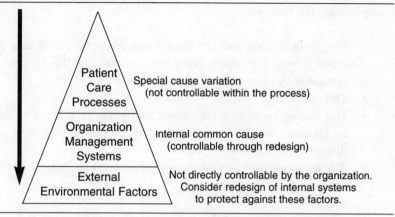

Patient Care Processes — Special cause variation (not controllable within the process)

Organization Management Systems — Internal common cause (controllable through redesign)

External Environmental Factors — Not directly controllable by the organization. Consider redesign of internal systems to protect against these factors.

Source: Joint Commission on Accreditation of Healthcare Organizations, 1998.

patients are frequently the result of common causes in organizational systems. For example, when individual physicians are admonished to avoid prescribing medications that lead to adverse drug-drug interactions, they may try very hard to do so. But the large number of possible drug-drug interactions and the constantly growing knowledge base in this area make it impossible for physicians to remember all of the possible interactions. Errors in memory will occur.

The individual physician prescribing process is likely to be improved only when it is seen as part of the larger medication use system that involves the pharmacy, nursing, and information management. One solution some organizations are using is a computer-based order entry system linked to a real-time expert system that provides feedback to the physician about potential adverse drug-drug interactions, enabling better-informed clinical judgment.[3] The solution to the problem has been found by addressing the common cause in the design of an organization's information management system, not by focusing on the special cause of error in the clinical process; that is, the physician's faulty memory.

For the health care organization, identification of a special cause for a clinical sentinel event should automatically lead to a search for the common cause(s) in the system(s) of which the process is a part. It is the larger system, not the process, that must be redesigned to reduce the likelihood of future sentinel events. Errors by individual physicians, nurses, and pharmacists should generate evaluations of the organizational systems in which they work and which support their work. These systems include the following:

- The credentialing and privileging processes for physicians and other licensed independent practitioners and the hiring and competency review processes for others
- The continuing education of staff
- The management of information, including facilitation of communication, accessibility of knowledge-based information, and linkage of information sources
- The measurement of system performance with respect to both processes and outcomes

It is the responsibility of the organization's management and clinical leaders to focus attention on systems that can be redesigned for improvement, rather than on processes and people who cannot control causes outside of themselves.

WHY PROCESSES FAIL

The characteristics of a high-risk process that tend to increase the risk of a process failure include the following:

- Variable input
- Complexity
- Inconsistency
- Tight coupling
- Human intervention
- Tight time constraints
- Hierarchical culture

Variable Input

The nature of the input to the process can greatly influence the reliability of the process, ultimately affecting the output (results) of that process. Specifically, a process that receives a variable input is more prone to dysfunction because the process itself must be modified to accommodate the input variation. In health care processes, the patient—who is the principal input—is highly variable.

Complexity

Complex processes are more prone to failure than simple ones. This seems obvious, yet we in health care have tended to design very complex processes, often of necessity given the nature of the work, but sometimes, it would seem, deriving satisfaction from the complexity itself and comforted by the assumption that nothing will go wrong. The more steps in a process and the greater their interdependence, the greater the complexity of the process. The more complex the process, the greater the chance of unanticipated and undesirable side effects and unrecognized long-term effects. Table 7-1 illustrates the problem.[4] For example, if the rate of error in each step is 1 percent (the "0.99" column in the table), then if there is only one step in the process, the likelihood of an error occurring in the process is 1 percent; if there are 25 steps, the likelihood of an error in the process is 22 percent; for 50 steps the likelihood of an error is 39 percent; and for 100 steps it is 63 percent!

Inconsistency

The tendency for a process to fail is also diminished in relation to the consistency with which it is carried out; that is, the degree to which it is standardized. Efforts in recent years to standardize health care processes through the introduction of practice parameters, protocols, clinical pathways, and so forth have been met with limited enthusiasm

Table 7-1.   Probability of Success in a Process

| Number of Steps | Probability of Success of Each Step | | | |
	0.95	0.99	0.999	0.9999
1	0.95	0.99	0.999	0.9999
25	0.28	0.78	0.98	0.998
50	0.06	0.61	0.95	0.995
100	0.006	0.37	0.9	0.99

among practitioners and are only slowly affecting the actual delivery of care. Achieving process consistency while retaining the ability to recognize and accommodate variation in the input (for example, the patient's severity of illness, comorbidities, other treatments, and preferences) is one of the major challenges to standardization in health care.

Tight Coupling

Given that a process is a series of actions, and recognizing that process failure very often occurs at the interface between the steps (actions) in a process, the characteristics of the relationships between actions become important. The relationship between the steps in a process is called *coupling* and is commonly described in terms of the tightness or looseness of the coupling.[5] A tightly coupled process is one in which the steps follow one another so closely that a variation in the output of one step cannot be recognized and responded to before the next step is under way. Thus the next step is dealing with an input (the output of the preceding, closely coupled step) that it may not have been designed to handle, and therefore may itself fail. This helps to explain the phenomenon of "cascade of failure" that often amazes the casual observer following a sentinel event. How could so many things have gone wrong at once? The answer, of course, is that the process was not designed to stop the chain of events once the initial failure occurred.

Human Intervention

Any process that depends heavily on the intellectual and physical intervention of humans will be more prone to failure than a process that does not have such dependency, such as automated activities. This is the case as long as things are going smoothly. Automated processes function better than human processes in a routine mode but often don't do as well when things start to go wrong.[6] Human judgment is still superior to a machine in dealing with an unanticipated contingency and adjusting the process to avoid harm. This distinction becomes important in defining the ideal roles of humans and technology, respectively, in complex processes. The strengths and weaknesses of each are, happily, complementary. The heavy dependence on human intervention in health care processes has recently led to a reconsideration of the meaning of "reliability" in this context. The traditional definition of reliability is *no variation*. Sutcliffe and Weick point out that a more practical definition for health care, as well as other high-risk activities that are heavily dependent on human intervention, would be "the ability to handle unforeseen situations in ways that forestall unintended consequences."[7] This requires a level of cognition and adaptation for which humans (so far) are superior to machines. It is often the *person* who "creates" safety for the individual patient in the health care process.[8]

Tight Time Constraints

Time truly is of the essence in so much of what we do, and especially so when dealing with acute illness or injury. Tightening the time constraints for human participation in a process tightens the coupling between steps, thus allowing less opportunity to identify, analyze, and respond appropriately (safely) to variation and thereby increasing the likelihood of failure. Health care processes often seem to have a certain inertia. Once in motion, they tend to keep moving, adding to the time pressure, further limiting opportunity to analyze a variation and plan an ideal response. Very loose time constraints can also increase the likelihood of failure, probably because of the human propensity for boredom or distraction.

Hierarchical Culture

The airline industry's crew resource management studies demonstrated clearly that the relationships among participants in a complex process, specifically the manner and degree to which they *communicate* with one another, can affect the overall reliability of the process.[9] Generally, a group of individuals interacting as a team, without constraints on communication based on rank or role, will function more reliably, both in stable and unstable situations, than a group that is constrained by hierarchical conventions such as, "The captain is always right; don't question the captain." The MedTeams project described by Risser and others in chapter 9 of this book illustrate how the lessons learned in the airline industry are now being applied to health care teams.

MEDICAL MANAGEMENT OF THE HEALTH CARE PROCESS

If the analogy used above is valid, then the approach to "healthier" (that is, safer) health care processes should follow the model for medical management: diagnosis, treatment, and follow-up (essentially the measure-assess-improve cycle). Proactive medical management of health care processes, as for health promotion and disease prevention, holds the promise of greater benefit for the resources consumed compared with simply reacting when something bad happens.

Diagnosis

A proactive approach to reducing risk means starting with a prospective risk assessment or diagnostic evaluation. Prospective risk assessment recognizes that things can and do go wrong and looks for those possibilities before they manifest themselves. What are the processes that pose the greatest risk to patients? How do those processes fail? What is it that most often goes wrong? Why? What other things might go wrong in the process? What does or might happen when such failures occur? And, ultimately, how could the patient be affected? These are the types of questions that are asked in Failure Mode and Effects Analysis (FMEA), an analytical method used for decades in engineering to identify and reduce hazards.[10] This technique examines a system's individual components to determine the variety of ways each component could fail and the effect of a particular failure on the stability of the entire system.

An important aspect of this prospective analysis is the determination of *why* certain failures might occur; that is, identifying the *root causes* of potential failure modes. The failure modes are not viewed as causes in themselves but as symptoms. In the case of an actual sentinel event, one of these failure modes might be the proximate or immediate cause identified at the start of the root cause analysis, perhaps a human error or equipment failure. Later in the analysis, we identify the underlying systemic factor(s) that enabled the proximate cause to occur. Using FMEA, people can identify weaknesses in a system design and predict what might happen as a result of those weaknesses. FMEA is especially useful in analyzing a new design or redesign, such as that which might be proposed following root cause analysis of a sentinel event. Another important application of this powerful analytical tool is in judging the effect of an uncontrollable external failure. For example,

What would be the impact on the organization's internal systems and, ultimately, its health care processes and outcomes if at midnight on December 31, 1999, the electrical power supply were suddenly interrupted and not restored for a week?

Realistically, FMEA cannot identify all possible failure modes or all of the effects of a failure (direct, indirect, or long-term), and it has limited efficacy in dealing with multiple-failure modes. No prospective risk assessment method, including FMEA, can guarantee uniformly good outcomes, but they can help to reduce the risk of bad outcomes when systematically applied.

Another related prospective analytical approach is called Fault Tree Analysis (FTA).[11] Whereas FMEA starts with the identification of all possible failures in the steps of a process or in the interactions between steps and then looks downstream for the effects and upstream for the causes, FTA starts with the identification of a potential effect—a hypothetical sentinel event, if you will—and works backward. A root cause analysis approach is used to pick the most likely process failures that could produce that effect. The analyst then works further back to identify the underlying systemic factors that could be modified to reduce the likelihood of that outcome.

A useful technique for testing a new process design is "worst-case" analysis. This involves a trial of the new process (on paper or using computer simulation) assuming the maximum likely variation in those factors that are generally uncontrollable, like the input to the process and the external environment in which the organization functions. For example, a hospital is designing a new emergency angiography unit. The facility, staffing, and procedural specifications are established. Then the worst-case scenario is hypothesized: What would happen if a 400-pound patient with active tuberculosis presented with a cold leg at 2 A.M. on a Sunday morning? Clearly an unlikely scenario, but such a hypothetical "stress testing" of the new process can unmask weaknesses that might otherwise go unnoticed until an equally unlikely situation actually occurred.

Determining the Treatment

When designing systems, engineers start with the premise that anything can go wrong, and they write volumes on analysis and prevention of potential failures. Health care professionals, on the other hand, tend to work from the premise that if they are competent in doing their jobs, nothing will go wrong (and if something does go wrong, it *could not* have been prevented). Given this attitude, health care professionals tend to write about failure only in retrospect. We do root cause analyses of what *went* wrong rather than prospective analysis of what *might* go wrong. Most of the psychological barriers to effective risk reduction disappear when the analysis anticipates rather than follows the failure. While the movement toward root cause analysis in response to sentinel events is necessary and will result in significant contributions to our understanding of medical errors, even greater advances will result from a cultural reorientation that acknowledges fallibility of systems, processes, and people. By encouraging prospective analysis of potential failures and supporting system redesign to minimize adverse outcomes, significant patient safety improvements can be realized.

An error—a failure in one or more steps of a process or in the transitions between steps—can lead to an undesirable outcome. Therefore, actions to reduce the likelihood of errors should be pursued whenever possible. The problem, of course, is that despite our best efforts to the contrary, things will still go wrong. The next challenge, then, is to further design our processes to accommodate this reality by building in safeguards to protect against a bad outcome even if an error occurs. Such treatment or protective design takes two forms: (1) preventing the error from reaching the patient, and (2) mitigating the effects of an error that reaches the patient.

Preventing the Error from Reaching the Patient If an error occurs in step 3 of a five-step process, and in step 4 someone recognizes the resulting variation in its expected input and (a) sounds an alarm and (b) interrupts the process, the error can then be corrected without an adverse result for the process as a whole (other than, perhaps, a minor delay while the error is being corrected). For example, a computerized medication order entry system may identify an unusual dose (perhaps the result of a misplaced decimal point), provide immediate on-line feedback to the ordering practitioner, and accept a corrected order, all before the patient receives the first dose. This represents a design that includes a means for recognizing an antecedent error, communicating the fact of the error, and modifying (temporarily halting) the process to deal with the error while protecting against an adverse outcome.

It is usually safer *not* to act (at least for a while) than to act incorrectly. Therefore, a process that is designed to detect failure and to interrupt the process flow is preferable to a process that continues on in spite of the failure. In a more general sense, we should favor a process that can, by design, respond automatically to a failure by reverting to a predetermined (usually safe) default mode. Very often it is simply enough to "pause" the process to allow for human intervention to assess and deal with the contingency. Modern software design with its warnings and required confirmations for high-risk actions such as "Delete all files? Y/N" is an example of a process interruption intended to minimize hasty actions that we may later regret.

In systems design, the term *redundancy* refers to a backup mode or a secondary means of accomplishing what the primary system was supposed to do if the primary system should fail. Requiring two nurses to independently check the label on a unit of blood against the patient's identification band is a type of system redundancy. To be maximally effective, the redundant systems should be independent of one another and not subject to the same external influences. If the systems are not independent of each other, the backup may be disabled by the failure of the primary system. If the primary and secondary systems are subject to the same external influences, the cause of a primary system failure would in all likelihood cause the backup (redundant) system to fail also. In this transfusion example, if both nurses check the blood container label against the same source document identifying the patient's blood type, and that document is in error, then both nurses will make the same mistake (for the same reason). To make matters worse, human redundancy, as in the transfusion example, is further complicated by the all-too-common assumption that the other person won't make a mistake (that is, the "nothing will go wrong" presumption) that results in a cursory and potentially inaccurate redundant check.

Even when systems are well designed, redundancy will always increase the complexity and, therefore, the risk of a failure. The failure of a redundant system will usually not be evident until the backup process is needed. Thus, redundant systems should be subjected to regular testing and maintenance. An obvious example is the necessary periodic testing of the emergency power supply for a hospital, a redundant system that ones hopes will not fail when it is needed.

Mitigating the Effects of an Error   The second form of protective design involves mitigating the effects of an error on the patient. For example, if a medication error has not been identified before the patient receives an incorrect dose, a well-designed system would ensure that the patient was monitored closely for the effects of the medication, any adverse effects would be quickly identified, and antidotes and other supportive medications and equipment would be readily available to mitigate the effects of the error.

Simplification We have often been admonished to K.I.S.S.—Keep it simple, stupid. A simple process is one that fully addresses the need without any extraneous parts or motion. But we must be careful not to confuse simplification with taking shortcuts. When people take short-cuts, even breaking safety rules at times, there are often no immediate consequences. Without consequences the perpetrators are relieved of the burden imposed by the rules and their behavior is thereby rein-forced. This kind of process simplification is obviously undesirable but may not be evident until revealed by a sentinel event unless the organi-zation conducts some type of prospective risk assessment.

Technology Finally, in selecting a treatment for a process found to be at risk of a failure, the role of technology must be carefully considered. Technology is a tool—actually an extensive, very powerful set of tools, but tools nonetheless. These tools should be seen as complementary to human intervention, not competitive. Computers and other technology lack the ability to make allowances for incomplete or incorrect infor-mation, an important requirement for dealing with complex situations.[12] Human judgment is still superior to a machine when dealing with an unanticipated contingency and adjusting the process to avoid harm. Technology is more effective than humans in enhancing process consis-tency and in receiving, storing, and processing information. Technology does not take shortcuts. It is not influenced by emotion. And it has the advantage of being a long-term improvement in contrast to risk-reduction strategies that, say, focus on staff retraining.

Implementing the Treatment

Once you've chosen the system redesign that is intended to reduce the chances that an error will occur or reach the patient if it does occur, or mit-igate the effect of an error if it does reach the patient, then it is time to con-sider how to best implement the change. In doing so, it is important to understand that the effect of a well-thought-out risk-reduction strategy may not always be what was intended. A "paper" analysis of the new design may be instructive and a lot less expensive than a premature implementation of a well-intended but faulty design. An example of a perfectly good "bad" idea was revealed during the planning for the Apollo moon landing. In an early model of the LEM (Lunar Excursion Module, later shortened to LM: Lunar Module), the design team recommended an innovative approach to vehicle stability on an unpredictably uneven landing surface. Risk assessment had identified the possibility of failure of one of the landing legs to fully extend prior to the controlled descent to the lunar surface. That was the *failure mode*. The *effects analysis* confirmed that such a (single-leg) failure would result in a "neutral stability" situation if the landing occurred on a perfectly smooth horizontal surface. "Neutral stability" means that although the vehicle might land in an upright position, even a slight irregularity of the surface, minor shift of weight distribution within the vehicle, or any number of other variables could cause the vehicle to fall over. This would be a mission-critical failure: there would be no way to launch the ascent stage of the vehicle back into lunar orbit if this presumed failure actually happened.

The solution: a fifth leg. With five legs evenly positioned around the periphery of the descent stage, a single leg failure would result in a stable situation—the center of gravity would remain within the outline of the remaining four legs. Ingenious. But wait. More legs means more legs could fail. What if two legs failed? As long as they were not adjacent to one another, the vehicle would still be in a stable situation, and the odds of two adjacent legs failing was felt to be vanishingly small. What a great idea!

But now let's look at the implications of this redesign. A fifth leg is quite problematic for engineers trying to design a vehicle whose propulsion systems require a high degree of symmetry in the payload they are moving. This is clearly a more complex design and therefore more prone to failure. It has other implications of great importance to a space vehicle. Legs are heavy. A 20 percent increase in the weight of the landing gear will require additional thrust capability from the descent stage engine. This means the engine may have to be heavier, and the liquid propellant supply will certainly have to be increased. This increased payload for the Lunar Module adds 10 times that weight to the Saturn launch vehicle in additional propellant requirements.

The lesson: things aren't always as good as they seem. It is particularly difficult to reject a clever solution to a vexing problem, especially when it is your own idea. But history is cluttered with good ideas gone bad. Thorough analysis and testing of any new or redesigned process or system will enhance its risk-reduction potential and decrease the likelihood of unintended consequences. The recommended approach is to first assess the potential effectiveness of a risk-reduction strategy on paper through application of failure mode and effects analysis, fault tree analysis, and other analytical techniques, with particular attention to potential side effects and long-term effects of the proposed process changes. Whenever possible, simulation testing should be considered. Simulation allows us to experience the implications of a redesign, albeit in a less complex environment without real risk to patients. It can reveal potential unanticipated side effects of variation in the process and, in the case of computer simulation, has the further advantage of allowing things to play out in compressed time to reveal long-term effects.

At some point the new or redesigned process will be implemented. Consider pilot testing as a prudent alternative to full-scale implementation. It can reveal much about the real-life effectiveness of the new process.

Follow-Up

Be sure to guard against the assumption that the absence of immediately obvious negative side effects means that the correct measures have been taken. Remember, the reason for making changes in the first place was to reduce the likelihood of an *infrequent* adverse outcome. To objectively conclude that the redesign is effective requires more than simply observing the absence of sentinel events.

For this reason, the measures of effectiveness should focus more on process than on outcomes. Objective measurement of the consistency, completeness, timeliness, and intermediate outputs of selected steps in the new process will provide greater assurances about the effectiveness of the changes and the suitability for full-scale implementation.

Finally, once the new or redesigned process is fully implemented, attention must be paid to maintaining the process and protecting it against the ravages of time. This will require documenting the new process, training staff in the new process and its redesigned system support, providing ongoing (preferably on-line) access to information about these new processes and systems, and continued monitoring of the new process. Examples of effectiveness measures for various processes are found in chapter 2 of this book.

Let us focus for a moment on documenting the new process. We all dislike documentation when there seems to be no immediate payback— documentation for documentation's sake. The risk is that failure to fully document a new or redesigned process can have its own unanticipated and unintended consequences. We need only to look at the nightmare (and costs) that the world is now experiencing as it attempts to hunt down every Y2K bug in our older, *undocumented* software programs. Failure to document these programs 20 years ago may mean, at the very least, some of us will not be able to withdraw money from an ATM machine on January 1, 2000. Process documentation is itself a proactive risk-reduction strategy not only for the short term (for example, to educate staff in the new process) but also for the long term in order to enable future root cause analyses of potential or actual sentinel events. Finally, where humans play a role in the process there will be a tendency to revert back to old ways. Appropriate technological support and, ideally, the involvement of leadership to induce a change in organization culture supportive of the new approach to safety will provide the greatest assurance of long-term success.

Figure 7-2 provides a checklist for organizing proactive risk-reduction activities. Recognizing that certain health care processes pose higher risks to patients than others, both in frequency and severity of adverse outcomes, it seems reasonable to focus these activities where the risks are greatest. Several suggestions for identifying such high-risk processes are offered in the figure, including a decision to implement a new service or modify an existing one. Integrating the risk-reduction activities described in this chapter into the design and redesign of health care processes will, over time, reduce the incidence of sentinel events in health care as it has in so many other fields. This checklist is provided as a tool to facilitate this integration.

CONCLUSION

Risk reduction strategies can be categorized and arranged according to the increasing likelihood of successful long-term effects, as follows:

1. Punitive actions directed at individuals
2. Counseling and retraining of individuals or groups
3. Process redesign

Figure 7-2. A Checklist for Proactive Risk-Reduction Activities

☐ Identify a high-risk process.
—History of adverse outcomes
—Identified in the literature as high risk
—Has several characteristics of a high-risk process (see page 184 of the text)
—New process
—Proposed redesign (such as in response to a sentinel event)
☐ Create a flowchart of the process as designed.
☐ Assess the actual implementation of the process (different locations, shifts, etc.).
☐ Identify where there is, or may be, variation in the implementation of the process; i.e., what are the failure modes?
☐ For each identified failure mode, what are the possible effects?
☐ Assess the seriousness (i.e., the "criticality") of the possible effects (e.g., delay in treatment, temporary loss of function, patient death).
☐ For the most critical effects, conduct a root cause analysis to determine why the variation (the failure mode) leading to that effect occurs.
☐ Redesign the process and/or underlying systems to minimize the risk of that failure mode or to protect the patient from the effects of that failure mode.
☐ Conduct a failure mode and effects analysis on the redesigned process with special attention on how the redesigned steps will affect other steps in the process and whether they will continue to do the beneficial things that the previous design could do.
☐ Consider simulation testing of the redesigned process.
☐ Consider a pilot test of the redesigned process.
☐ Identify and implement measures of the effectiveness of the redesigned process.
☐ Implement a strategy for maintaining the effectiveness of the redesigned process over time.

---

4. Technical system enhancement
5. Cultural change

Unfortunately, the ease with which these types of changes can be successfully implemented is in reverse order of their efficacy.

Risk-reduction strategies that include punitive actions directed at individuals and counseling and retraining of individuals or groups are the quickest to enact. Unfortunately, these are the least effective in achieving long-lasting change. Process redesign and technical system enhancement are far more labor-intensive risk-reduction strategies, but the likelihood of sustainable improvements is far greater.

Health care organizations need not wait for sentinel events to occur in order to reduce process errors. We can start today. We know a great deal already about where the risks are in health care, and we are learning more every day. The tools are available for analyzing high-risk processes. The techniques for designing safe processes are also known, waiting only to be adapted to health care. It is time for a reality check. We are not perfect. We must design accordingly.

References

1. *Random House Unabridged Dictionary*, 2d ed. (New York: Random House, 1993).

2. H. Gitlow et al. *Tools and Methods for the Improvement of Quality* (Homewood, IL: Richard D. Irwin, Inc., 1989), pp. 163, 171.

3. D. W. Bates et al. "Effect of Computerized Physician Order Entry and a Team Intervention on Prevention of Serious Medication Errors," *JAMA* 280, no. 15 (1998): 1311–16.

4. D. M. Berwick. "Taking Action to Improve Safety: How to Increase the Odds of Success," conference presentation, Enhancing Patient Safety and Reducing Errors in Health Care, Rancho Mirage, CA (November 1998).

5. C. Perrow. *Normal Accidents: Living with High-Risk Technologies* (New York: Basic Books, 1984), pp. 89–100.

6. J. T. Reason. *Managing the Risks of Organizational Accidents* (Aldershot, UK: Ashgate Publishing, Ltd., 1997), pp. 45–46.

7. K. M. Sutcliffe and K. E. Weick. "The Reduction of Medical Error Through Systemic Mindfulness," conference presentation, Enhancing Patient Safety and Reducing Errors in Health Care, Rancho Mirage, CA (November 1998).

8. R. I. Cook. "Two Years before the Mast: Learning How to Learn about Patient Safety," conference presentation, Enhancing Patient Safety and Reducing Errors in Health Care, Rancho Mirage, CA (November 1998).

9.   R. L. Helmreich et al. "Preliminary Results from the Evaluation of Crew Resource Management Training: Performance Ratings of Flight Crews," *Aviation, Space, and Environmental Medicine* 61 (1990): 576–79.

10. J. M. Juran and A. B. Godfrey. *Juran's Quality Handbook*, 5th ed. (New York: McGraw-Hill, Inc., 1999), pp. 19.25–19.26, 48.30–48.31.

11. Ibid.

12. J. T. Reason. *Managing the Risks of Organizational Accidents.*

8

Reducing Errors through Work System Improvements

Patrice L. Spath, BA, ART

I n the mid-20th century, with the discovery of sulfonamides, penicillin, and other antibiotics, antitubercular drugs, and the polio vaccine, people began to think that medicine had the potential to successfully treat all disease.[1] In the 1950s and 1960s an explosion of new medical technology further fueled society's optimism over conquering disease. In this climate the errorless imperative evolved in which both health professionals and society demanded that mistakes not be made.[2] While the errorless imperative is a nice ideal, increases in medical technology have actually heightened the chance of error because health care practitioners must learn highly specialized skills. The decline in infectious diseases has been countered by an increase in such chronic conditions as heart disease, cancer, and respiratory disorders. These health problems tend to require more technology and complex medical interventions that, in turn, intensify the risk of error.[3] The fact remains that health care practitioners are only human and not perfect, and there are no guarantees that mistakes won't be made and patients won't occasionally be injured.

Errors can occur in all aspects of health care services. During the diagnostic phase practitioners can fail to order indicated tests, misread lab results, or fail to act on the results of diagnostic findings. During the treatment phase a technical error can occur in preparation or performance (for example, miscalculation of dose, delivery of treatment to the wrong patient, or mishap during surgical procedure). Treatment can be mistakenly delayed, or inappropriate care can be provided. During the preventive phase of health care, practitioners can inadequately monitor patients during prophylactic treatments or provide insufficient follow-up. Communication errors and equipment failures can occur at any time.

Over the past 50 years, behavioral scientists have studied the nature, varieties, and causes of human error in hopes of discovering what can be done to reduce errors or mitigate their effects. Students of human performance believe that all people err on occasion and that although a human is usually involved when accidents occur in a professional setting such as health care, the causes of the error are likely to be out of the individual's control.[4] Thus, the personal approach to error management—individual training and punishment—has not proven to be a long-lasting patient safety improvement strategy. The balance of scientific opinion clearly favors finding and eliminating the error-producing factors in tasks, the workplace, and the organization.[5,6] Accident prevention requires an understanding of what is happening and why it is happening. Armed with this situational understanding, practitioners can then formulate appropriate task, workplace, and organizational improvements.

Anesthesiology has already begun to apply this situational approach to error management, with resulting improvements in ergonomics, operating room layout, monitoring interfaces, and other systemwide refinements. Anesthesia-related deaths are now at about 1 in 200,000 to 300,000, down from approximately 2 in 10,000 a decade ago.[7] Some of these situational changes in anesthesia administration came about as a result of retrospective accident investigations.[8,9] An increasing number of proactive efforts are also under way to find and correct error-producing factors before an accident occurs.[10]

Although accident investigation techniques have been used for many years in private industry, there has been little written about development of postaccident prevention recommendations. For example, only one of the 13 chapters in *Root Cause Analysis: A Tool for Total Quality Management* describes how to develop solutions.[11] The 1,992-page Management Oversight and Risk Tree (MORT) *Accident/Incident Investigation Manual* only contains two paragraphs about making recommendations.[12] Ludwig Benner, Jr., a long-time safety consultant and currently the executive vice president of Events Analysis, Inc. (Oakton, Virginia), has observed that about 90 percent of the person-hours in an accident investigation are typically invested in determining what happened and preparing a report of those findings versus about 10 percent in recommendation development. He suggests this ratio should be more in the range of a 50-50 to 60-40 split.[13]

Conventional wisdom suggests that a well-done root cause analysis will result in the development of good improvement recommendations. However, this does not always occur. The purpose of this chapter is to familiarize health care practitioners with the general error-reduction strategies and specific process changes that have proven to be success-ful in both industrial and health care settings. Several general work sys-tem improvements designed to reduce or mitigate the effects of human error are contained in the first section of this chapter. Because the processes involved in medication administration are risk prone, a spe-cial section is devoted to a discussion of process improvements that have been shown to reduce the likelihood of errors. With the growing array of complex medical devices, equipment-related accidents are on the rise. Tips on how to reduce these types of errors are included in the section on equipment. One of the more popular error-reduction strate-gies is automation. While automating tasks can potentially diminish common slips or mistakes, automation itself introduces a different class of hazards into the health care workplace. The last section of this chap-ter is devoted to a discussion of these risks and what to do to minimize automation-related errors.

The recommendations included in this chapter are not intended to represent the entire universe of improvement choices. However, the suggestions should serve as an effective starting point when developing redesign recommendations during an accident investigation or for proactive error management purposes. Readers are cautioned against indiscriminate adoption of any process change. The unique circum-stances of each organization must be taken into consideration, as well as the impact on collateral processes. Haphazard process improvement is tantamount to tampering, and tampering can lead to chaos with an eventual increase in errors.[14] Experience in the nuclear power industry has shown that some preventive "fixes" actually played a major role in causing subsequent accidents.[15]

ERROR MANAGEMENT STRATEGIES

Researchers in human factors analysis have been dealing with the causes and effects of human errors since the 1940s. Originally applied to the design of increasingly complex military aircraft cockpits, the study of human factors is being effectively applied to such diverse settings as nuclear power plants, NASA spacecraft, and health care. Armed with a better understanding of the cause of human errors, people hope to redesign systems and processes to enhance human performance and reduce errors and accidents.[16] High-reliability industries, such as aviation, air traffic control, and nuclear power, learned long ago the fallacy of relying on human perfection to prevent accidents. Like health care, these industries believe in training, rules, and high standards, but they don't rely on them. They look to their systems.[17]

If the health care industry is to improve patient safety, systems and processes must be designed to be more resistant to error occurrence and more accommodating of error consequence. To achieve this goal, we must first understand the error environment and where errors are most likely to occur. Information for this evaluation can be based primarily on observation (by walk-throughs or talk-throughs) or experience (examination of past incidents and errors). Once the error environment is understood, organizations can better match expected error-causing situations with appropriate redesign solutions. It is impossible to eliminate all error risk; however, process improvements that preferentially deal with error occurrence first and error consequences second are recommended.

Two types of process redesign can affect error occurrence. The first is known as *error elimination*, in which the process is changed so an error is impossible to make. An example is the anesthesia machine that was redesigned so that the connector for the oxygen tank could not fit into the nitrous gas tank, thus making it impossible for the anesthesiologist to make a connection error. At times, deleting the error-prevalent task from the process can subsequently eliminate mistakes. For example, in 1996 it was discovered that hospital nurses were making significant errors in the administration of concentrated potassium chloride solutions.[18] Many hospitals subsequently removed this medication from the floor stocks as suggested by the U.S. Pharmacopeia, thereby taking the nurse out of the process entirely.

If error elimination is not possible or feasible, then the next best choice is to *reduce error occurrence* through process redesign. Because error elimination is difficult, error reduction is the most common objective for many of today's process improvements in health care. In the example above, removing the nurse from the process of mixing parenteral solutions that contain potassium chloride may have eliminated the chance of nursing error, but delegating the admixture tasks to pharmacists does not prevent them from making a mistake. Controls would need to be built into the pharmacy processes to reduce the likelihood of error.

The third approach to process redesign is to *eliminate the consequences of errors*. Given that mistakes will occasionally happen, the process can be designed to catch errors before eventual patient harm occurs. An example of a task intended to eliminate error consequences is the final system check done by anesthesiologists before using any anesthetic apparatus, ventilator, breathing system, or monitor. This process step is employed to detect and correct such problems as misfilled oxygen cylinders, contamination of liquid oxygen reservoirs, incorrect connections within the machine, and other device malfunctions.[19]

If errors and consequences cannot be completely eliminated, consider process improvements intended to *reduce the effect of errors*. This may be achieved through application of process design features that prompt actions to mitigate the consequences of an error. For example, laboratory technicians have been trained to immediately flush their eyes with water if they've been splashed with a toxic substance. Unfortunately, few patient care processes have similar automatic interventions designed to mitigate the consequence of errors. Perhaps, as suggested by Lori B. Andrews, lead researcher in a recent study of medical adverse events, "We've misled ourselves into thinking that errors are infrequent, so we don't incorporate the potential for error as part of the ongoing process."[20]

Several general work system improvement principles have come out of human factors studies. These principles, listed in figure 8-1, suggest how people's working conditions can be changed to eliminate or reduce error occurrence.[21–26] These process improvements can also be useful in eliminating the consequence of errors or mitigating the effects of an error.

Simplify the Process/Reduce Hand-Offs

Simple processes are easier for people to understand and errors are easier to recognize and correct before an accident occurs. Many errors come from slips in transfers of materials, information, people, instructions, and/or supplies. Processes with fewer hand-offs are at less risk for mistakes. In an effort to improve the administration of heparin, caregivers at Promina Gwinnett Health System in Lawrenceville, Georgia,

Figure 8-1. Work System Improvement Principles

- Simplify the process/reduce hand-offs.
- Reduce reliance on memory.
- Standardize.
- Improve information access.
- Use constraints and forcing functions.
- Design for errors.
- Adjust work schedules.
- Adjust the environment.
- Improve communication.
- Decrease reliance on vigilance.
- Provide adequate safety training.
- Choose the right staff for the job.

began stocking standard heparin solutions and boluses on the nursing units. After this process change, the time elapsed between placing an order for heparin and hanging an IV bag with the correct dose decreased from 202 to 90 minutes.[27] In 1993 Memorial Hospital in Jacksonville, Florida, set out to improve timely administration of thrombolytic therapy for patients diagnosed with a myocardial infarction. The project team discovered that its current process of triaging emergency patients with chest pain contained up to 16 different steps, all of which occurred prior to the patient's even being seen by a physician. By eliminating some of the hand-offs in the triage process, the team was able to reduce the number of steps to just five. Other processes, such as EKG ordering, were also simplified. Ultimately, the emergency department at Memorial Hospital was able to achieve a reduction in door-to-needle time for thrombolytic therapy from an average of 69.30 minutes to an average of 18.39 minutes.[28]

Reduce Reliance on Memory

With the seemingly unlimited information needed to perform a particular job, people's memory limits can easily be exceeded. Easy-to-use information retrieval systems can help to reduce errors caused by memory overload. Checklists, protocols, clinical pathways, preprinted physician orders, and computerized decision aids are common examples of point-of-care reminders that can reduce people's reliance on memory. Practitioners at William Beaumont Hospital in Royal Oak, Michigan, use several point-of-care reminders as part of their interdisciplinary outcomes management initiative.[29] Pathway project teams, cochaired by a physician and a nurse or a professional from another department conduct a review of current literature and industry best-practice standards. Each pathway project results in three documents:

1. *Clinical Practice Guidelines.* This document outlines the treatment decisions for those aspects of patient care for which evidence or consensus is required. The guidelines are based on current research and, where research is lacking, physicians' personal observations.
2. *Physician Order Sheet.* All items that require physician orders are on one sheet (see figure 8-2). Separate medication order sheets may be developed for those patient groups that require numerous complicated medication/IV orders.
3. *Clinical Pathway.* This document is used by the multidisciplinary team to coordinate patient care activities. It also serves as a tool for nursing documentation, taking the place of the problem list or plan of care. The pathway includes common patient problems and expected outcomes and recommended nursing and clinical support service interventions.

The clinical practice guidelines and physician orders at William Beaumont Hospital are approved by the affected medical staff departments and the medical care evaluation committee. The clinical pathway is approved by a work group of the hospital nursing practice committee. The director of pharmacy and, when appropriate, an infectious disease consultant also approve the pathway content.

In its analysis of the causes of medication errors, the Institute for Safe Medication Practices (ISMP) has found that, at times, preprinted order sets can contribute to mistakes. To reduce the possibility of errors, institutions are encouraged by the ISMP to have some methods and rules in place to evaluate and use order forms. The following suggestions offered by the ISMP are applicable to any type of point-of-care reminder tool:[30]

- Do not use preprinted orders unless all disciplines are involved in the process of developing, reviewing, and finally approving the forms.
- Do not allow orders if they don't coincide with hospital policy (for example, "renew all previous orders" is not permitted in many hospitals).

Figure 8-2. Physicians' Order Sheet

ATTENTION PHYSICIAN:	This preprinted form is available to facilitate patient care. Order items by checking the box in front of the item and/or completing the blanks where necessary. This is not for pharmacy orders. If additional items are needed, add them on the standard Doctors Order sheet.

1. Admit to: ☐ Emergency Care Observation Unit
   ☐ Medical Care Unit
   ☐ Cardiac Progressive Care Unit
   ☐ Critical Care Unit
   ☐ Other _____

2. Condition: _____

3. Allergies: _____

4. Vital Signs: ☐ per unit protocol   ☐ orthostatic vital signs every shift

5. Activity: ☐ Bathroom privileges with assistance
   ☐ _____

6. Nursing Treatments: ☐ Intake & output
   ☐ Daily weight
   ☐ Teaching per clinical pathway
   ☐ Cardiac monitor/telemetry monitor service
   ☐ Other _____

7. Laboratory Tests: ☐ CK-MB Q 8 hours (total 3) ☐ _____
   ☐ Hgb Q 6 hours × 2   ☐ _____
   ☐ _____

8. Diagnostic Studies: ☐ EKG in AM   ☐ STAT EKG with chest pain
   ☐ 2D Echo re: _____ (if not done in EC)

9. Respiratory Care: ☐ O$_2$ per respiratory protocol

10. Diet: ☐ Cardiac Diet ☐ _____ ☐ _____ cal ADA

11. Consultation:
    Pulmonary re: embolus workup ☐ Dr._____ re: _____
    GI re: rule-out bleed   ☐ Dr._____ re: _____
    Cardiology re: EPS or tilt table ☐ Dr._____ re: _____
    Psych consult   ☐ Dr._____ re: _____
    ☐ Dietitian, re: _____ ☐ Continuing Care re: _____

12. CPR Status Order: ☐ Full CPR (Call CPR team)
    ☐ No CPR (CPR team will not be called, no chest compressions will be initiated by unit staff in the event of cardiopulmonary arrest.)

_____
   Attending Physician Signature

13. ☐ Old charts to floor

Physician Assistant Signature	Date	Time	Physician Signature	Dr. Page No.	Date	Time
Noted by Unit Secretary	Date	Time	Noted by R.N.		Date	Time

Source: William Beaumont Hospital, Royal Oak, MI. 1999. Reprinted with permission.

- Avoid ambiguous statements such as "unless allergic, give . . ." because this type of statement transfers clinical and legal responsibility from the prescriber to others down the line. Develop and use a uniform system to indicate orders that should or should not be followed.
- Use generic names on forms and specify reason for administration wherever possible. For single-source items, brand names should also be included. Make sure no forbidden abbreviations or dangerous dose designations are used on the forms. Each hospital should have a list of these.
- Require the dose per m2 or dose per kg for all chemotherapy and pediatric orders when a calculated dose must be entered.
- Do not include a list of drugs to choose from because it's too easy to choose the wrong item (for example, vincristine has been confused with vinblastine).
- Force entry of the daily dose and number of days for any multiple-day regimens.
- Express doses by metric weight (for example, 5 mg) rather than by number of tablets, mL, and so on unless the drug isn't measured by weight (like milk of magnesia).
- Avoid coined names like "magic mouthwash" or "banana bag" because they may be misunderstood by people unfamiliar with them.
- Enhance readability by using fonts and print styles that are of professional quality.
- Proper spelling and spacing is important (for example, propranolol20 mg is easily misread as propranolol 120 mg).
- Lines on the back of any order form are unnecessary and may hide decimal points or portions of a number or name. Tell the printer to leave them off.
- Print a tracking number and revision date on the form to ease replacement.
- Review all preprinted orders every two or three years or when protocols change.

Standardize

If a task is done the same way every time—by everyone—there is less chance for error. Areas in which unnecessary variation may be found include drugs, equipment, supplies, work processes, and the location of equipment and supplies in a patient care unit or on a code cart. Standardizing the abbreviations that can be used when ordering medications is an important step toward decreasing medication errors. Physicians are used to using their own abbreviations and styles when writing orders, thus creating many opportunities for errors when these orders are interpreted by pharmacy staff. In hopes of reducing such mistakes, the physicians and pharmacists at Baptist Medical Center in Columbia, South Carolina, developed order-writing guidelines for the ICU. The guidelines are posted on the front of each patient's chart. The pharmacy found that nonconforming orders dropped from an average of 15 percent before the process change to 9 percent after the change.[31] Caregivers at Methodist Hospital in Indianapolis were able to reduce the incidence of occipital pressure ulcers from cervical spine immobilization from 19 to 0 in an 18-month period after standardizing mobilization products and patient care protocols.[32]

Improve Information Access

Good decisions require good information. People must have ready access to relevant and complete information or faulty decisions can occur. In a 1997 study of the use of an "evidence cart" during patient rounds at the University of Oxford in England, researchers found that making evidence quickly available to clinicians increased the extent to which evidence was sought and incorporated into patient care decisions.[33] Better communication of information is the goal of the recommendations of the American Academy of Orthopaedic Surgeons for eliminating wrong-site surgery.[34] According to its advisory statement, the incidence of wrong-site surgery can be reduced by having the surgeon's initials placed on the operative site using a permanent marking pen and then operating through or adjacent to his or her initials. The patient's records should also be available in the operating room. Many hospitals are actively including patients in this communication loop, with patients encouraged to initial the surgical site themselves or mark "NO" on the limb not requiring surgery.[35]

Not only must information be accessible, it must also be up-to-date. The Food and Drug Administration is aware of four cases of hemolysis that have occurred since 1996 during or following plasmapheresis when

Albumin (Human) 25 percent was diluted to a 5 percent final protein concentration using Sterile Water for injection. The hospital pharmacies in these cases apparently relied on information contained in the 1994 edition of Trissel's *Handbook on Injectable Drugs* that was revised in the 1996 edition.[36] The importance of having up-to-date references is emphasized.

Use Constraints and Forcing Functions

Constraining functions, such as the "Are you sure?" prompt that follows hitting the delete key in a computer program, make it more difficult to commit errors. Forcing functions, such as being unable to start your car when in reverse gear, are an effective method for error-proofing processes. An example of a constraining function that was shown to reduce medication errors in a residential care is described by Chappell and others.[37] Researchers found that caregivers who used prefilled 7-day medication dispensers to administer residents' medications had fewer omission errors than those who used the traditional prescription bottle method of dispensing. Caregivers using prescription bottles committed 113 omission errors during the 3-week study period, compared with only 21 omission errors by the group using dispensers. Researchers also observed that the medication dispensers prompted caregivers to order prescription refills in a more timely manner than caregivers using the traditional bottle method. The medication dispenser acted as a constraint that reduced errors.

Computer-based recognition procedures and disposable blood bag combination locks are two forcing functions currently being tested in blood transfusion services. It is hoped that these process changes will eliminate transfusion errors caused by failure to comply with traditional unit-recipient identification protocols.[38]

Design for Errors

Design systems that encourage error detection and correction before an accident occurs. At Fairview Health Services in Minneapolis, pharmacists are empowered by the medical staff to modify ordered doses of certain drugs based on patient status. After instituting this process change, the appropriateness of benzodiazepine dosing for patients over the age of 65 went from 25 percent to 100 percent in a two-week time period. Similar medication dosing improvements have occurred in other drug classes.[39] Pharmacists are provided with medical staff–approved protocols and are allowed to automatically intervene when a physician orders an inappropriate medication dose.

All high-risk processes should include double-checks. A recent theophylline overdose event involved an infant in the neonatal intensive care unit who inadvertently received 11 mL, not the 11 mg, of aminophylline that was ordered. The nurses in the unit in which this incident occurred were solely responsible for preparing doses taken from stock without being checked by at least two individuals. Double-check systems are critically important, especially with "high-alert" drugs where the consequences of errors are great and even minor dose miscalculations could prove disastrous.[40]

Adjust Work Schedules

Practices such as failing to provide a sufficient number of staff members for the job (increasing workload) and frequently altering work shifts of employees (increasing fatigue) can ultimately lead to errors in human performance. Experts at the 1996 National Association of Pharmacy Boards Health Law Officers conference in Savannah recommended that to ensure safe medication dispensing, not more than 10 to 20 prescriptions should be filled per hour by a pharmacist.[41] Recent studies are beginning to substantiate an inverse relationship between nurse staffing levels in hospitals and adverse events.[42,43] The long hours that medical residents are expected to remain on duty are said to affect the quality of patient care.[44]

Adjust the Environment

Human factors engineers have long recognized the error-producing factors in work environments; for example, noise, poor lighting, glare-producing surfaces, heat, clutter, electrical interference, humidity, and moisture. Staff members working in less-than-ideal situations are more likely to make errors. Conduct worksite analyses to identify human performance problems related to workstation design, workplace layout, equipment, supplies, and procedures. The results of these analyses can be used to identify possible hazards and develop solutions for eliminating or controlling them.

Reducing hazards in the environment can also directly influence a reduction in patient accidents. For example, obtaining functional wheel locks for beds, improving the lighting, repositioning call lights, and adding assistive devices such as raised toilet seats have been shown to reduce the rate of falls among nursing home residents.[45]

Improve Communication

To reduce mistakes, avoid indirect communication among the work team and cut down on the number of communications per task. Often, determining the most appropriate patient care action requires effective sharing of information among the health care team and collective decision making. In 1992, following questions raised by the work of the American Society of Anesthesiologists' Difficult Airway Task Force, the Division of Critical Care Anesthesia at Johns Hopkins Medical Center undertook a project designed to improve communication concerning patients who have a known history of difficult airway/intubation.[46] Their hope was to establish a uniform way that physicians can be informed of critical information about past incidents. Several aspects of this project involved patients. A highly visible temporary bracelet is placed on any patient identified as having a difficult airway or intubation, and a special label is placed on the hospital chart. Select patients are recommended for and enrolled into the permanent Medic Alert Foundation International emergency medical ID system. The patient is given a wallet card containing his or her medical record and a highly visible permanent bracelet or necklace to attract the attention of health care personnel should the patient fail or be unable to relate his or her airway problem.

In chapter 9 of this book Risser and others describe techniques for improving how health care team members establish and maintain a common understanding of patient and operational issues through communication improvements.

Decrease Reliance on Vigilance

When people are expected to devote too much of their attention to a problem or situation, they are apt to become forgetful or complacent in their vigilance. An example of a simple, yet successful reminder system was implemented at Promina Gwinnett Health System. In studying the process of heparin administration it was noted that when a patient's prothrombin time was too high, the heparin was placed on hold and the nurse had to remember to start the heparin again in one hour. The restart did not always occur on time when the nurse's attention became focused on some other task. The nurses now carry pocket timers to remind them to resume the heparin infusion in exactly one hour.[47]

Involving the patient and family in vigilance tasks can also help reduce errors. When patients understand the medications, treatments, and tests they are receiving they can be active partners with the health care team to help prevent errors. The American Academy of Orthopaedic Surgeons encourages patient involvement to reduce wrong-site surgeries. The American Society of Hospital Pharmacists (ASHP) has long advocated that health care providers encourage patients to take an active role in their drug use by questioning and learning about their treatment regimens. Generally, if patients are more knowledgeable, anxieties about the uncertainty of treatments can be alleviated and errors in treatment may be prevented.[48] The American Academy of Pediatrics (AAP) reaffirmed these recommendations in their 1998 policy statement on prevention of medication errors. In this statement, the AAP suggests that physicians should speak with the patient or caregiver about the medication that is prescribed and any special precautions or observations that should be noted. The AAP also encourages nurses to listen when a patient questions whether a drug should be administered and, if appropriate, double-check the medication order.[49]

The Institute for Safe Medication Practices has developed consumer tips for taking medicines safely, which include recommendations for how people can work with their caregivers to overcome problems that are known to lead to medication errors. Many organizations have incorporated the recommendations from the ISMP into their patient education programs. Figure 8-3 is an excerpt from the patient handbook at Memorial Hospital in Towanda, Pennsylvania. This portion of the handbook tells patients and their families how they can help in eliminating medication errors. Some people in the hospital may be unable to take an active part in making sure the correct medication is administered. For these patients, the ISMP has created red stop-sign stickers that boldly state, "STOP—Check Nameband." These can be affixed to patient gowns as a visual reminder to verify patient identity before administering medications or initiating any treatment.[50] In some instances, a friend, relative, or patient advocate can assume a vigilance role.

Many hospitals are partnering with patients and families to reduce the risk of infant abductions. The National Center for Missing and Exploited Children recommends that parents be provided with written security instructions and educated on department routines, such as tests, feedings, and visiting hours. It is also recommended that parents be instructed to never leave their infant out of direct line of sight even for a moment and never release their infant to anyone without the proper identification.[51] Down East Community Hospital in Machias, Maine, has developed a family education guide for infant security (figure 8-4) that is shared with parents, if possible, during prenatal education classes. The guide asks parents to partner with hospital staff in protecting the newborn child and provides important safety information.

Figure 8-3. Patients' Role in Medication Usage

Medications

Medications are often an integral part of your therapy during hospitalization. We at Memorial Hospital would like to ensure that your medications are administered safely and accurately. You can play an active role in this process by participating as a member of your health care team. When medicines are brought to you, please:

- Show your identification wrist band to the nurse or therapist so that he or she can establish that the medication is meant for you.
- Inform your nurse of any allergies or reactions you have experienced in the past. You will be provided with a red wrist band listing the medications or products to be avoided. Please check that the information on the band is correct and show this bracelet to the nurse or therapist each time you are given a drug.
- Become familiar with the medications you are receiving. Question the professional as to the name of the drug and why you are receiving it. Ask if there are any side effects to expect. We are more than happy to teach you.
- Most important, never hesitate to speak up if you sense there is a problem. If you don't recognize a drug, or if a nurse is administering the same medication you received ten minutes before in a different department, we will thank you to call it to our attention. Errors are often detected by well-informed patients. Your awareness assists us in our quest for excellence.

Figure 8-4. **Sample Family Education Guide for Infant Security**

Your baby's safety is a priority at Down East Community Hospital. Although infant kidnapping has never occurred here and in general is rare, Down East Community Hospital takes precautions to be sure your baby is protected. You can help by following these important steps.

1. *Become familiar with the hospital staff who will work in the mother/baby unit.* Two nurses are present to care for you and your baby. Nursing shifts usually change at 7 A.M. and 7 P.M. At those times the nurse you know will introduce the new nurses to you. <u>The nurses you know and your physician are the only persons who have any reason to take your baby anywhere.</u> Housekeeping staff, lab and dietary persons, and other people may be in to deliver flowers or mail. <u>These persons have no reason to take your baby anywhere. If you have any questions about any of these people, press your call light and your nurses will assist you.</u>

2. *Never leave your baby alone or unsupervised in the room.* If you leave your room or go into the bathroom, ask a family member to watch your baby or send your baby to the nursery. We allow you maximum access (rooming-in) with your baby. If you wish to take a nap, place the bassinet near the head of your bed, away from the door, or send your baby back to the nursery.

3. *No one is allowed in the nursery without an invitation by the staff.*

4. *Never allow anyone to walk with your baby in the hallway.* <u>Always use the rolling crib to take your baby from the nursery or return her/him to the nursery.</u>

5. *Your baby can only be taken from the nursery by you or dad. You, dad, or your family can request that your baby be brought to your room anytime.*

Other steps the staff takes to safeguard your baby include:

- We place matching ID bands on you and the baby at birth, take footprints of the baby and your fingerprints, check your baby over soon after birth, and write down any unique features.
- We keep cord blood samples for blood testing.
- There are electronic eyes on the nursery doors.
- We limit access of staff and visitors to your baby and to the nursery.
- We do not give any information about you to telephone callers without your permission.
- We will transfer the calls to you or your family whenever possible.

TOGETHER, we can make your stay with us safe and secure.

Source: *Family Education Guide for Infant Security,* Down East Community Hospital, Machias, ME. © 1999. Reprinted with permission.

Provide Adequate Safety Training

Make employees aware of the potential hazards relevant to their job and the given strategies for avoiding them. If faced with an unsafe situation, staff members must know what steps to take and they must be empowered to act. After a patient died of a massive fluid overload following hysteroscopy surgery to remove a uterine fibroid, practitioners at Beth Israel Hospital in New York found that the surgeon had failed to heed several warnings from the circulating nurse and scrub nurse about the patient's lack of fluid output.[52] One of the policy changes made subsequent to the incident is that the circulating nurse must notify the surgeon and the anesthesiologist when input of the distention medium exceeds output by 1,500 mL. The surgeon is expected to terminate the procedure as soon as hemostasis can be obtained. Failure by the surgeon to terminate the procedure is grounds for summary suspension. If this policy had been in place prior to the patient's surgery, the death may have been avoided.

Likewise, staff must be prepared to act in case of a life-threatening emergency. Thomsen and Bush studied management strategies for patients who experience an adverse reaction to radiographic contrast materials.[53] Although the incidence of reactions is low (0.2 to 0.4 percent of patients receiving nonionic low-osmolar contrast media, 1 to 2 percent of patient receiving ionic high-osmolar contrast media), the authors suggest that radiologists and their staff remain sufficiently trained and prepared to take immediate action should a reaction occur. Periodic drills or rehearsals are especially important for those situations that rarely happen to ensure that practitioners maintain their skill proficiencies.

Choose the Right Staff for the Job

For any job or task, it is important to identify people with the abilities necessary to perform the job safely. Staff members must also be adequately trained in the competencies necessary to perform the job and their readiness confirmed prior to work execution. Organizations should have written policies and procedures that include competency standards for each patient care area and a method for measuring individual performance against these competency standards. Facilities should have mechanisms for rapid deployment of competent personnel when any labor-intensive event occurs, for example, multiple admissions or discharges or an emergency health crisis for an individual patient.

Float staff should be assigned only to those areas for which they have received orientation. Likewise, the float staff must have demonstrated competency to care for patients in that area; otherwise they should not be given full responsibility for a patient assignment. For example, a nurse who has not been oriented to, and demonstrated the ability to manage, a ventilator should not be assigned responsibility for the care of a patient on a ventilator.

Multiple Work System Improvements Are Needed

Human errors can occur for a number of reasons. Errors can be directly attributed to system and process design and environmental and personnel factors. To reduce and/or eliminate human error occurrence in a risk-prone process, more than one work system improvement is necessary. For example, the occurrence of errors due to faulty communication cannot be entirely eliminated through improved training or optimal staffing. As a consequence, a variety of work system improvements must be enacted to minimize the occurrence and limit the consequences of human error. There is no quick one-time fix that is likely to be effective.

The recommendations for process changes that have been distributed by the Joint Commission are an example of how comprehensive the system redesigns might need to be in order to reduce adverse patient events. In reviewing sentinel events involving the death of patients while in restraints, the Joint Commission and those organizations that have experienced this type of occurrence have offered many suggestions for preventing and reducing restraint deaths. These recommendations are listed in figure 8-5.

The administration of medication is a very complex process and, as such, requires a multifaceted approach to addressing errors. Human error in this high-risk process is best addressed with overlapping error occurrence prevention and reduction and consequence prevention and reduction initiatives. Such a layered defense strategy is characteristic of the error management activities found in the nuclear industry and other complex technical systems.

Figure 8-5. Strategies to Help Reduce the Risk of Restraint-Related Deaths

---

- Redouble efforts to reduce the use of physical restraint and therapeutic hold through the use of risk assessment and early intervention with less restrictive measures.
- Revise procedures for assessing the medical condition of psychiatric patients.
- Enhance staff orientation/education regarding alternatives to physical restraints and proper application of restraints or therapeutic holding.
- Consider age, sex, and gender of patients when setting therapeutic hold policies.
- Revise the staffing model.
- Develop structured procedures for consistent application of restraints.
- Continuously observe any patient that is restrained.
- If a patient must be restrained in the supine position, ensure that the head is free to rotate to the side and, when possible, the head of the bed is elevated to minimize the risk of aspiration.
- If a patient must be restrained in the prone position, ensure that the airway is unobstructed at all times (for example, do not cover or "bury" the patient's face). Also, ensure that expansion of the patient's lungs is not restricted by excessive pressure on the patient's back (special caution is required for children, elderly patients, and very obese patients).
- Never place a towel, bag, or other cover over a patient's face as part of the therapeutic holding process.
- Do not restrain a patient in a bed with unprotected split side rails.
- Discontinue use of certain types of restraints, such as high vests and waist restraints.
- Ensure that all smoking materials are removed from patients' access, including access from family and friends.

Source: *Suggested Strategies for Preventing and Reducing Restraint Deaths,* Joint Commission on Accreditation of Healthcare Organizations. © 1998. Reprinted with permission.

PROTECTING AGAINST MEDICATION ERRORS

Researchers estimate that more than 30 million doses of medication are given daily in U.S. hospitals, nursing homes, and extended care facilities. There are many complexities of medication administration that make it an error-prone process. First, there are currently more than 8,000 drugs available for physicians to order. At a minimum, three people are involved in medication administration: the doctor who writes the order, the pharmacist who dispenses the medication, and the nurse who gives the medication to the patient. There are usually a considerable number of individual process tasks that occur between the time of medication ordering until administration. All of these factors add up to a high probability of mistakes in the process of medication delivery, with some mistakes having the potential to cause patient injury.

The Institute for Healthcare Improvement (IHI), founded in 1991 by Donald M. Berwick, MD, is working to improve health care quality by fostering collaboration among organizations. Using systems analysis tools, collaborative participants apply commonly used safety principles and methods to make changes and improvements at their organizations in a particular area. In March 1997, the IHI announced key findings from their collaborative of 42 health care organizations nationwide that, at that point, had worked together for one year to reduce and prevent medication errors. Many of these suggestions, listed below, illustrate the application of one or more of the work improvement principles described earlier in this chapter.[54,55]

- Create clear guidelines and standards for writing medication orders.
- Develop preprinted medication order forms, where possible, listing the most commonly prescribed drugs with selected dosages, frequencies for administration, and times for administration.
- Avoid using abbreviations such as "u" for units, "pcn" for penicillin, "QD" for every day, "QID" for four times daily, and "QOD" for every other day.
- Eliminate the use of trailing zeros—use 2mg instead of 2.0mg.
- Always use leading zeros—use 0.125mg instead of .125mg.
- Order medications by "mcg," "mg," or "g" strength when possible (for example, indicate Tylenol 650mg instead of Tylenol 2 tabs or Roxanol 20mg instead of Roxanol 1cc).
- Eliminate the use of "Resume Previous Orders." Insist upon full rewrites of existing orders or require physicians to sign off on computer-generated records of their previous medication orders.
- Automatically reduce doses in the pharmacy for patients who have poor kidney or liver function.

- Ensure safe handling of lethal drugs. The administration of potassium in a concentrated form is a common fatal error. Take the following actions in order to reduce errors:
  - —Remove potassium from the floor stock, completely eliminating the chance of an accidental concentrated infusion. Have the pharmacy premix diluted forms of potassium.
  - —Institute double-checks when administering any concentrated dose by IV.
  - —Highlight critical information on medications by using special labeling.
- Establish standard drug administration times to reduce the chance of omissions.
- Ensure that all medication rooms are identical throughout the hospital (that is, store all items in the same place in each room).
- Standardize the number of dosing options (for example, use only 2 concentrations of narcotics, heart medications, heparin, and so on) to reduce the chance of incorrect dosages.
- Develop a protocol establishing clear guidelines for prescribing and administering any complex dosing regimen (for example, heparin and insulin are two commonly used medications for which the dose varies throughout the day, depending on lab results).
- Improve chemotherapy safety. Chemotherapy involves complex dosing and scheduling, using drugs in combination and involving a number of crucial details in administration. Standardizing the process helps reduce the chance for error.
  - —Develop preprinted orders with detailed listings of dose limits for chemotherapy drugs—maximum per dose, per course, and per lifetime.
  - —Create and train a special chemotherapy team that is responsible for all ordering and administration of chemotherapeutic drugs (strong familiarity with new drugs and complex procedures reduces the possibility of error).
  - —Require medication orders to be written prior to admission and lab work to be done in advance as much as possible to allow ample time for double-checking all protocols.
- Improve access to information. Make critical information readily available. Place all information regarding patients, medications, and equipment closest to where it is to be used (for example, place order-writing standards on the patients' charts,

have translation charts of brand and generic drug names posted next to the narcotics cabinet, and so on).

- Use color-coded wrist ID bands on patients with known drug allergies.
- Put allergy information automatically on all medication order forms.

Medication errors occurring in the outpatient environment have not received the same study attention as those occurring in hospitals and nursing homes; however, these errors can also be a patient safety risk. In a one-year review of 8.5 million visits that elderly patients made to a physician, researchers found that in approximately 5 percent of the visits, one or more inappropriate medications were prescribed for the patients.[56] Because medication errors are a liability concern, many malpractice insurance companies disseminate error-reduction suggestions to their participants. Based on its analysis of medication-related claims, Medical Mutual Insurance Company of Maine developed and distributed the recommendations shown in figure 8-6.

EQUIPMENT

Equipment problems are a common cause of untoward events. Leape found that nearly 4 percent of hospitalized patients sustained disabling injury associated with medical treatment, and that "technical complications" were the third most common type of adverse events (behind drug complications and wound infections).[57] Hart reported that equipment problems were the most common source of ICU adverse incidents, most of which affected the cardiovascular and respiratory systems.[58] Today's health care practitioner must know how to operate a wide array of complex machines. With the relentless progress of technology, practitioners will continue to be challenged by the ever growing number of devices. That's why managing equipment safety issues should be a regular part of every health care facility's error management strategy. Ensuring practitioner competency in the use of machines and equipment is an ongoing challenge. A 1991 Food and Drug Administration survey revealed that many anesthesiologists at that time clearly did not have a thorough understanding of their anesthesia machines.[59]

Figure 8-6.   Tips for Reducing Medication Errors in the Physician's Office

- All patient information sheets should have the allergy section filled in. If the patient denies any allergies, the standard abbreviation NKA (no known allergies) should be used. A blank entry can lead one to believe that the question as to allergies was never asked.
- If patient information sheets are not used, notations regarding allergies should uniformly be displayed in a conspicuous area in the file.
- Allergies to medications should be periodically updated. In addition, inquires should be made as to use of over-the-counter (OTC) drugs as well as prescriptions from other health care providers. One of the best times to do this is when there is a medication renewal or when a new medication is prescribed. However, at a minimum, the patients should be asked about their use of OTC medications or prescriptions from other health care providers annually. Questions regarding the effectiveness and usage of the medication, as well as appearance of side effects, are also important considerations during these conversations.
- All discussions with the patient regarding allergies, side effects, dosage, special procedures for taking (with meals or milk), or other issues should be documented by the involved staff member. If a medication instruction sheet or adverse reaction information is given to the patient, this should also be documented.
- Each time a medication is ordered, review the patient's medication history for contraindications, allergies, or excessive numbers of prescriptions or refills. If a patient is noncompliant in appropriately using prescription medications, explore the possible reasons with the patient. It could be something as simple as a misunderstanding of how the drug should be taken.
- If it is the policy of your office that the office staff call in routine prescription renewals (e.g., oral contraception, antihypertensive meds, etc.), it is important that there be written protocols identified for each specific renewal. For example, antihypertensives will only be provided if a blood pressure has been obtained within the last _____ days and falls within _____ range.
- If a nurse or other staff member is employed to triage requests for medications, all prescriptions resulting from those assessments should be approved by the physician before being given to the patient/family or called in to the pharmacy. In addition, staff should document information as to the pharmacy called, date, individual receiving the order, etc. for all telephone orders placed to the pharmacy.
- If the office is dispensing samples for use as a trial, be sure the sample has the instructions for use clearly identified on the bottle or carton. If not, put on a label describing the dose, route, and frequency. Be sure to document that samples were provided as well as how many total doses were given.
- If medication samples are kept in the office, they should be out of sight in nonpatient areas.
- It is a good idea to rotate the medication sample stock to avoid outdated medications.

(Continued on next page)

Figure 8-6. (Continued)

- Inspection logs should be maintained on all medications stored in your office. If controlled substances are kept in the office, there should be a written policy regarding compliance with state and federal regulations, security, and disposal. Also, access to controlled drugs should be limited to certain office employees.
- All practitioners should know the drugs they are prescribing, including correct dosage, contraindications, and side effects of the medication. Drugs unfamiliar to you should never be prescribed. Not only do unfamiliar drugs enhance the potential for patient injury, but also they can lead to medication errors and a potential professional liability claim.
- The emergency drug cart should be stocked with appropriate medications that are clearly marked. In offices where treatment is rendered to children, drugs should be maintained in pediatric doses.
- A medication flow sheet should be used to track medications. Not only does this give the practitioner a concise history, it allows for quick identification of: excessive renewals, potential problems with drug dependency, problems with drug efficiency, drug interactions, contraindications, and allergies.
- Lab values for medications requiring additional assessment (coumadin, theophylline, plaquenil, etc.) can be added to the medication flow sheet as a reference as well as a reminder.

Source: Medical Mutual Insurance Company of Maine. © 1999. Reprinted with permission.

Equipment can contribute to adverse events by either directly causing the accident or contributing to human errors that cause accidents. Even if equipment malfunction is the direct cause of the accident, malfunctions can often be traced back to human error (poor training or maintenance). The recent equipment-related event described below illustrates the human component of equipment failures.[60]

A 40-year-old man underwent uneventful aortic valve replacement surgery and was transported to the intensive care unit (ICU) and placed on a Bourns Bear 2® ventilator. Within 40 seconds of initiation of mechanical ventilation, the patient became hypotensive (BP = 60/40 mmHg). Initial urgent evaluation focused on a presumed bleeding source or possible cardiac or aortic valve complication. Fortunately, following arrival and evaluation by an experienced respiratory therapist and attending intensivist, it was noted that the ventilator was malfunctioning. The patient was immediately removed from the ventilator and hand ventilated with 100% FiO_2 until he could be placed on another ventilator.

Analysis of the incident revealed that the ICU personnel routinely worked with only two models of ventilators and were very comfortable with trouble-shooting problems rapidly in those devices. The Bear 2® ventilator was a back-up and only used in situations of intense ICU activity and maximal patient census. Few of the ICU staff had experience using this equipment. Thus, the contributing factor in this equipment failure was staff lack of training and education necessary for maintaining expertise and proficiency in a rarely used piece of equipment. The exhalation value malfunction that occurred in the Bear 2® ventilator is a known problem, but only to those familiar with the equipment. The latent failure in this event was the organization's decision to use old equipment for back-up purposes without ensuring that staff proficiency was maintained for these rarely used devices.

In evaluating the circumstances surrounding accidents or near misses involving equipment, investigators have identified common situations or problems that existed prior to the incident:[61]

- Staff training has been slow and arduous.
- Only a few staff members seem to be using the device.
- Staff tends to modify the equipment and takes shortcuts.
- Staff refuses to use the device.
- Staff finds installation of accessories difficult, confusing, or overly time-consuming.
- Alarms and batteries often fail.
- Incorrect accessories sometimes are installed.
- Parts often become detached.
- Equipment displays are difficult to read or understand.
- Equipment controls are poorly located or labeled.
- Alarms are difficult to hear or distinguish.
- Alarms are very annoying.
- Equipment operation is illogical and confusing.

If one or more of these device-related situations is known to exist in your organization, it should be viewed as a warning signal. Be sure to investigate and correct the problem before an untoward incident occurs. In the Bear 2® ventilator equipment malfunction, only a few personnel knew how to use the device. Fortunately, those people were available and acted quickly. However, the situation could have been avoided altogether if the early warning signs had prompted further investigation and action.

AUTOMATION

Of the 301 health care organizations responding to the 1998 information systems survey sponsored by *Modern Healthcare*, many indicated that they have, or are in the process of, implementing automated systems that will potentially improve patient safety. Within a short time, 76 percent expected to have computerized order entry, 57 percent will have networkwide systems that allow access to patient information (including history), and 43 percent will have clinical decision-support workstations.[62] Only 18 percent of the respondents indicated they already had, or were in the process of implementing, expert systems. These automated systems contain rules and decision algorithms that incorporate knowledge and judgment about the health problem at hand and alternative tests and treatments. These decisions are built into the expert-based system in the form of "if-then" rules as well as scoring algorithms, such as: "If the patient's potassium is less than 3.0 mEq/dl and the patient is on digoxin, then the clinician should consider ordering potassium supplementation."[63]

Safety-Critical Features May Still Be Missing

Efforts to computerize processes such as medication prescription and administration have the potential for reducing some types of errors. A recent study found that computerized physician order entry reduced preventable adverse drug events by 55 percent.[64] In another study, the use of a computer-based prompting system enabled anesthesiologists to more accurately select correct drugs and dosages during an emergency situation.[65]

Unfortunately, not all of today's automated medication-prescribing systems contain safety-critical elements, such as linkage of laboratory and pharmacy computer systems and adequate screening for interactions and patient allergies.[66] After completing a survey of 309 hospital pharmacy computerized systems, the Institute for Safe Medication Practices put together the following statistics:[67]

- Only 4 (1.3 percent) of the 307 systems tested were able to detect *all* unsafe orders presented in the field test.
- Only about 38 percent of respondents' systems detected lethal overdoses of both cisplatin (204 mg for a 26 kg child) and vincristine (3 mg for a 2-year-old).
- Eighty-seven percent did not detect an excessive antibiotic dose for a patient with renal impairment (tobramycin 120 mg IV q8h for a patient whose creatinine clearance was 10 mL/min).

As more organizations invest in expert systems that link all components of the patient's health record, some of these safety problems will be resolved.

Automation works best when it effectively "pauses" the process when an error is detected. It is usually safer to *not* act (at least for a while) than to act incorrectly. Automated systems should pause to allow for human intervention to assess and deal with the contingency. Reason suggests that, to be an effective error-reduction tool, reminders should (when possible) block further progress until the necessary step is completed.[68] However, most respondents to the ISMP survey indicated that their systems require no staff action (such as entering a password) to ensure that warnings are acknowledged. Thus, each warning can be bypassed simply by pressing a function key and may be overlooked by those working under pressure.

Errors Enabled by Automation

There is little doubt that technology will make significant contributions to the safety of health care processes. On the other hand, the addition of automation may create the opportunity for errors that had not been possible in the past or increase the chance of previously existing errors to occur. An example of a type of error that has been enabled by the newer highly automated aircrafts is one involving a gross navigational deviation caused by a data entry error. In the 1995 crash of American Airlines flight #965 in the Columbian Republic, investigators believe that wrong information entered into the airplane's automated navigational system ultimately resulted in the aircraft's hitting the side of a mountain.[69] According to investigators, this error would have been less likely to occur in older, less automated navigation systems. The airline industry is currently working to identify and understand the errors that will be encountered in new aircraft and how they can be successfully controlled. The health care industry should be undertaking similar investigations of newly automated systems.

There is speculation in the airline industry that the use of automation may make task management more difficult for flight crews, possibly leading to unsafe conditions. Task management refers to the process by which humans manage their available sensory and mental resources in a dynamic, complex, safety-critical environment in order to accomplish multiple tasks that are competing for their limited quantity of attention.[70] Health care practitioners working in highly complex or rapidly changing environments (like intensive care units, emergency departments, operating rooms, emergency medical services, and so on) are much like the flight crews on commercial airlines. These people must prioritize the tasks they perform because they do not possess the necessary resources to simultaneously execute all the tasks that demand their attention. Preliminary studies in the airline industry suggest that although task management errors occurred in both advanced and traditional technology aircraft, these errors seem to appear more frequently in the advanced technology aircraft.[71] Cook's study of anesthesiologists' use of new computer technologies in the operating room suggest that task management may become increasing important as health care adopts more advance automated systems.[72] When conducting new system training programs for clinicians, it will be important to heighten their awareness about the potential for task management errors.

In their detailed analysis of errors that can occur in a variety of automated control systems, including aviation, anesthesia, nuclear power plants, and space flight, Sarter and Woods have identified a number of human factors problems.[73,74] Automated systems can do the following:

- Increase demands on users' memory
- Cause users to be uncertain as to where and when they should focus their attention
- Make it difficult for users working in teams to share the same situational awareness

- Impair mental models of the system
- Increase workload during high-demand periods
- Limit the users' ability to develop effective strategies for coping with task demands
- Increase stress and anxiety
- Increase the potential for confusion (with many possible levels and types of automated systems)

Although these are not insurmountable problems, it is important that health care practitioners realize that automation may create new errors that are potentially more serious than those we are seeking to avoid. Vigilance and continued analysis of the cause of errors is important.

CONCLUSION

In a perfect world there would be no errors, and the operations of a health care facility would be under complete control at all times. There would be no unplanned, undesirable events and no accidents, incidents, or inefficiencies. Unfortunately, such perfect control does not exist in any organization that I know of. Every human action taken in the provision of health care services is an opportunity for error. An action may be a visible act, such as raising the patient's bedrails; an internal process, such as reading the patient's health record; or even a lack of activity, such as omitting the procedural step of checking the patient's allergy history.

A review of human error analysis in the health care literature reveals a growing number of studies that define types of human errors and methods for analyzing errors. Many of these studies are based on previous human factors work in other complex industries. In contrast, very little solution-oriented literature is found; for example, strategies for linking these human error reduction principles to existing process improvement efforts or summaries of design solutions that have demonstrated success in reducing or mitigating the effects of human errors in medicine. This literature void is likely to change as groups such as the National Patient Safety Foundation, the Veterans Health Administration, the Institute for Healthcare Improvement, the Anesthesia Patient Safety Foundation, and others further their efforts in patient safety research.

The problem of errors in health care is now recognized as a major health-quality issue. It will not disappear from public concern. A body of research on the prevalence and etiology of medical error has emerged, informed in part by the experience of the aviation and nuclear power industries and by students of human factors engineering.[75] Learning more about the error environment in your organization is far more important than determining who made the mistake. Focus improvements on the way things are done on the job, rather than the individuals doing the job. Corrective action should first be sought through modification of systems and processes, not through placing blame.

References

1. S. Y. Fagerhaugh et al. *Hazards in Hospital Care: Ensuring Patient Safety* (San Francisco: Jossey-Bass, 1987), pp. 3–4.

2. Ibid., p. 137.

3. Ibid., p. 5.

4. J. T. Reason. *Human Error: Causes and Consequences* (New York: Cambridge University Press, 1990).

5. D. Meister. "Human Error in Man-Machine Systems," in S. Brown and J. Martin, eds., *Human Aspects of Man-Made Systems* (Milton Keynes: The Open University Press, 1977), pp. 299–324.

6. J. T. Reason. *Human Error*, p. 130.

7. Joint Commission on Accreditation of Healthcare Organizations, "Sentinel Events: Approaches to Error Reduction and Prevention" (book excerpt), *Joint Commission Journal on Quality Improvement* 24, no. 4 (April 1998): 179.

8. J. B. Cooper, R. S. Newbower, and R. J. Kitz. "An Analysis of Major Errors and Equipment Failures in Anesthesia Management: Considerations for Prevention and Detection," *Anesthesiology* 60, no. 1 (1984): 34–42.

9. V. Chopra et al. "Reported Significant Observations During Anesthesia: A Prospective Analysis Over an 18-Month Period," *British Journal of Anaesthesia* 68, no. 1 (1992): 13–17.

10. M. E. PatJ-Cornell. "Risk Analysis Model Targets Anesthesia Incidents," *Anesthesia Patient Safety Foundation Newsletter* 7, no. 2 (Summer 1992): 13–20.

11. P. F. Wilson, L. D. Dell, and G. F. Anderson. *Root Cause Analysis: A Tool for Total Quality Management* (Milwaukee, WI: ASQ Quality Press, 1993).

12. W. G. Johnson. *Accident/Incident Investigation Manual*, 2d ed., DOE/SSDC 228-45/27 (Washington, DC: U.S. Department of Energy, 1985).

13. K. M. Hendrick and L. Benner. *Investigating Accidents with STEP* (New York: Marcel Dekker, 1987).

14. M. D. Sloan. *The Quality Revolution and Health Care* (Milwaukee, WI: ASC Quality Press, 1991), p. 29.

15. J. T. Reason. *Managing the Risks of Organizational Accidents* (Aldershot, Eng.: Ashgate Publishing Co., 1997), p. 52.

16. D. L. Welch. "Human Error and Human Factors Engineering in Health Care," *Biomedical Instrumentation and Technology* 31, no. 6 (November/December 1997): 627–31.

17. L. L. Leape. Congressional testimony to the Subcommittee on Health of the Committee on Veterans Affairs (October 8, 1997).

18. "Intravenous Potassium Predicament," *USP Quality Review* 22, no. 56 (October 1996).

19. Association of Anesthetists of Great Britain and Ireland. *Checklist for Anaesthetic Apparatus* (London: The Association of Anaesthetist of Great Britain and Ireland, March 1997).

20. M. Blecher. "Accident Scenes," *Hospital & Health Networks* 71, no. 10 (1997): 46–48.

21. L. L. Leape et al. *Breakthrough Series Guide: Reducing Adverse Drug Events* (Boston: Institute for Healthcare Improvement, 1998), pp. 80–83.

22. L. L. Leape. "Reducing Adverse Drug Events," conference presentation, National Forum on Quality Improvement in Health Care, Orlando, FL (December 9, 1998).

23. D. M. Berwick. "Taking Actions: Leading the Reduction of Error," conference presentation, Examining Errors in Health Care, Rancho Mirage, CA (Ocober 1996).

24. American Society of Health-System Pharmacists. "Top-priority Actions for Preventing Adverse Drug Events in Hospitals: Recommendations of an Expert Panel," *Am J Health Syst Pharm* 53, no. 7 (1996): 747–51.

25. L. L. Leape. "Preventing Medical Injury," *Quality Review Bulletin* 19, no. 1 (1993): 144–49.

26. L. L. Leape et al. "Systems Analysis of Adverse Drug Events," *JAMA* 274 (1995): 35–43.

27. L. Leape et al. *Breakthrough Series Guide*, p. 38.

28. M. Dagher. "Using Process Improvement Techniques to Manage Patient Outcomes," in P. Spath, ed., *Medical Effectiveness and Outcomes Management: Issues, Methods, and Case Studies* (Chicago: American Hospital Publishing, Inc., 1996), pp. 207–20.

29. P. L. Spath. "The Future of Collaborative, Path-Based Practice," in S. S. Blanchett and D. L. Flarey, eds, *Health Care Outcomes: Collaborative Path-Based Approaches* (Gaithersburg, MD: Aspen Publishers, Inc., 1998), pp. 19–31.

30. M. Cohen. "Preprinted orders," *ISMP Medication Safety Alert* 3, no. 8 (1997): 1.

31. L. Leape et al. *Breakthrough Series Guide*, pp. 28–29.

32. J. Powers. "A Multidisciplinary Approach to Occipital Pressure Ulcers Related to Cervical Collars," WWW document: http://best4health.org/html/tools/tool3_abstract.htm (October 24, 1999).

33. D. L. Sackett and S. E. Straus. "Finding and Applying Evidence During Clinical Rounds: The 'Evidence Cart,'" *JAMA* 280, no. 15 (1998): 1336–38.

34. American Academy of Orthopaedic Surgeons Advisory Statement, WWW document: http://www.aaos.org/wordhtml/papers/advistmt/wrong.htm (October 1997).

35. "Patient Involvement: The Right Idea to Prevent Wrong Site Surgery. Stops Drug Errors Too!" *ISMP Medication Safety Alert* 3, no. 24 (1998): 2.

36. "Hemolysis and Renal Failure Associated with Inappropriate Use of Sterile Water to Dilute 25% Albumin Solution," *Medical Bulletin of the Food and Drug Administration* 28, no. 1 (summer 1998): 1.

37. H. W. Chappell, C. Dickey, and M. DeLetter. "The Use of Medication Dispensers in Residential Care Homes," *Family and Community Health* 20, no. 10 (1997): 10.

38. B. Wenz, F. Mercuriali, and J. P. AuBuchon. "Practice Methods to Improve Transfusion Safety by Using Novel Blood Unit and Patient Identification Systems," *Am J Clin Pathol* 107, no. 4 (April 1997): Suppl1, S12–16.

39. S. Meisel. "Reducing Adverse Drug Events," conference presentation, National Forum on Quality Improvement in Health Care, Orlando, FL (December 9, 1998).

40. "Safety Briefings," *ISMP Medication Safety Alert* 4, no. 4 (1999): 2.

41. North Carolina Board of Pharmacy. "Pharmacy Workload," board statement, WWW document: http://www.ncbop.org/workload.htm) (March 26, 1997).

42. C. Kovner and P. J. Gergen. "Nursing Staffing Levels and Adverse Events Following Surgery in U.S. Hospitals," *Image: Journal of Nursing Scholarship* 30, no. 4 (1998): 315–21.

43. M. A. Blegen, C. J. Goode, and L. Reed. "Nurse Staffing and Patient Outcomes," *Nursing Research* 47, no. 1 (January 1998): 1, 43–50.

44. J. Greene. "Residents Say Long Hours Hurt Patient Care," *American Medical News* 42, no. 9 (1999): 1, 30–31.

45. W. A. Ray et al. "A Randomized Trial of a Consultation Service to Reduce Falls in Nursing Homes," *JAMA* 278, no. 7 (1997): 557–62.

46. L. J. Mark. "'Medic Alert' System for Difficult Airway Is Subject of National Communication Effort," *Anesthesia Patient Safety Foundation Newsletter* 7, no. 2 (summer 1992): 17–18.

47. L. Leape et al. *Breakthrough Series Guide*, p. 38.

48. American Society of Hospital Pharmacists. "ASHP Guidelines on Preventing Medication Errors in Hospitals," *Am J Hosp Pharm* 50, no. 2 (1993): 305–14.

49. American Academy of Pediatrics, Committee on Drugs and Committee on Hospital Care. "Prevention of Medication Errors in the Pediatric Inpatient Setting," *Pediatrics* 102, no 2 (1998): 428–30.

50. To obtain a small supply of these stickers, send a self-addressed stamped envelope to the Institute for Safe Medication Practices, 300 W. Street Rd., Warminster, PA 18974-3231.

51. National Center for Missing and Exploited Children. *For Healthcare Professionals: Guidelines on Prevention and Response to Infant Abductions* (Arlington, VA: NCMEC, 1998).

52. P. Patterson. "Fine Levied After Hysterectomy Death," *OR Manager* 14, no. 12 (1998): 6.

53. H. S. Thomsen and W. H. Bush, Jr. "Adverse Effects of Contrast Media: Incidence, Prevention, and Treatment," *Drug Safety* 19, no. 10 (1998): 313–24.

54. The Institute for Healthcare Improvement. "The Quest for Error-Proof Medicine," *Drug Benefit Trends* 9, no. 6 (1997): 18, 23, 27–29.

55. L. Leape et al. *Breakthrough Series Guide.*

56. R. R. Aparasu and S. E. Fliginger. "Inappropriate Medication Prescribing for the Elderly by Office-Based Physicians," *Ann Pharmacotherapy* 31, no. 7–8 (1997): 823–29.

57. L. L. Leape et al. "The Nature of Adverse Events in Hospitalized Patients," *New Engl J Med* 324, no. 6 (1991): 377–84.

58. G. K. Hart et al. "Adverse Incident Reporting in Intensive Care," *Anaesth Intens Care* 22, no. 5 (1994): 556–61.

59. D. E. Lees. "Pre-operative Check-list Revisited," *ASA Newsletter* 55, no. 8 (August 1991): 9–11.

60. R. C. Prielipp, K. Lewis, and R. C. Morell. "Ventilator Failure in the ICU: DJjB Vu All Over Again," *Anesthesia Patient Safety Foundation Newsletter* (1998).

61. D. Sawyer. *Do It By Design: An Introduction to Human Factors in Medical Devices* (Washington, DC: Center for Devices and Radiological Health, Food and Drug Administration, 1996), p. 32.

62. J. Morrissey. "Y2K: Ready or Not," *Modern Healthcare* 29, no. 8 (February 22, 1998): 68.

63. R. F. Gibson and B. Middleton. "Health Care Information Management Systems To Support CQI," in S. D. Horn and D. S. P. Hopkins, eds., *Clinical Practice Improvement: A New Technology for Developing Cost-Effective Quality Health Care* (New York: Faulkner & Gray, 1994).

64. D. W. Bates et al. "Effect of Computerized Physician Order Entry and a Team Intervention on Prevention of Serious Medication Errors," *JAMA* 280, no. 15 (1998): 1311–16.

65. A. J. Schneider et al. "'Helper': A Critical Events Prompter for Unexpected Emergencies," *J Clin Monit* 11, no. 6 (1995): 358–64.

66. G. D. Schiff and D. Rucker. "Computerized Prescribing: Building the Electronic Infrastructure for Better Medication Usage," *JAMA* 279, no. 13 (1998): 1024–29.

67. "Over-reliance on Pharmacy Computer Systems May Place Patients at Great Risk," *ISMP Medication Safety Alert* (February 10, 1999).

68. J. T. Reason. *Managing the Risks of Organizational Accidents*, p. 98.

69. "Preparing for Last-Minute Runway Change, Boeing 757 Flight Crew Loses Situational Awareness, Resulting in Collision with Terrain," *Flight Safety Foundation Accident Prevention* 54, no. 7/8 (1997): 1–13.

70. K. Funk et al. "Agenda Management: Understanding and Facilitating the Management of Flightdeck Activities," WWW document: http://www.engr.orst.edu/~funkk/AMgt/amgFull.html#ctm (February 1999).

71. J. R. Wilson and K. Funk. "The Effect of Automation on the Frequency of Task Prioritization Errors on Commercial Aircraft Flight Decks: An ASRS Incident Report Study," conference presentation, Second Workshop on Human Error, Safety and System Development, Seattle, WA (April 1998).

72. R. I. Cook and D. D. Woods. "Adapting to New Technology in the Operating Room," *Human Factors* 38, no. 4 (1996): 593–613.

73. N. B. Sarter and D. D. Woods. "Mode Error in the Supervisory Control of Automated Systems," conference presentation, Human Factors Society 36th Annual Meeting, Atlanta, GA (October 1992).

74. D. D. Woods et al. *Behind Human Error: Cognitive Systems, Computers and Hindsight. State of the Art Report* (Dayton, OH: CSERIA, Wright-Patterson Airforce Base, 1994).

75. L. L. Leape. Congressional testimony to the Subcommittee on Health of the Committee on Veterans Affairs (October 8, 1997).

9

A Structured Teamwork System to Reduce Clinical Errors*

Daniel T. Risser, PhD
Robert Simon, MEd, EdD
Matthew M. Rice, MD, JD, FACEP
Mary L. Salisbury, RN, MSN

Teamwork is defined as a "cooperative effort by members of a group or team to achieve a common goal."[1] More than a decade of research in aviation has shown that effective teamwork is critical to flight safety.[2-5] Both the armed services and commercial aviation organizations have standardized training systems in place for teamwork. What the aviation industry has found is that teamwork training reduces the risk that crews will make a fatal error or permit a fatal string of errors to unfold because the crew failed to communicate, coordinate, and check each other. The training has significantly improved teamwork, resulting in saved aircraft and lives. For Army aviation, teamwork training has meant over 20 percent improvement in mission performance, over 40 percent reduction in safety-related task errors, and an estimated annual savings of 15 lives and $30 million.[6,7]

There is an increasing awareness in the health care community that teamwork training can have similar patient safety benefits. Shifts in caregivers' attitudes and beliefs, such as those listed below, have prompted the health care community to examine the various accident reduction methods used in industries such as aviation.

---

*Copyright © 1999 Dynamics Research Corporation. All rights reserved.

- The realization that all humans are fallible and that even the most diligent and conscientious clinicians will make mistakes frequently simply because they are human.[8-16] The willingness to face such human limitations and seek solutions that are attentive to these limitations has historically been missing in health care.[17-19]

- The realization that one caregiver's error can often be anticipated and prevented or corrected by another caregiver if the clinical work environment can accept and actively embrace the idea of mutual real-time monitoring for errors by peers. Peer monitoring is beginning to be seen positively as a safety net that protects both the patient and the caregiver. Permitting, perhaps even asking, other caregivers to regularly check one's actions is a dramatic attitude change for the health care community.[20]

- The realization that the health care delivery system is complex and poorly designed. This poor design, in combination with medicine's complexity, dramatically increases the risk of error.[21,22] The medical community has just begun to recognize that problems exist in the ways caregivers coordinate services.[23,24] Better solutions will only come from a better understanding and better design of the care processes.[25-28]

- The realization that caregiver training is too narrow. While health care professional education does an excellent job of teaching clinical skills, attention to coordination skills has been missing.[29,30] The teaching of teamwork skills and team concepts to improve care delivery has been dramatically missing.[31]

There is a strong potential that teamwork training for emergency care providers will have benefits that are comparable to aviation. Functionally, the emergency care world has much in common with aviation. It requires effective and often rapid coordination of groups of technical professionals to execute critical technical tasks, demands appropriate sequencing and timely execution of tasks, often demands quick decision making using incomplete information, and imposes high standards of performance and high levels of responsibility and stress on the professionals involved. Just as crews, passengers, and aircraft are placed in danger when aircrew teamwork fails, patients suffer when emergency caregivers improperly coordinate care or fail to help each other prevent clinical errors. Such errors, in the most extreme forms, permanently

injure patients and lead to deaths. In a less extreme form, errors use-
lessly consume time and resources and slow patient recovery.[32] Both
forms of error provide good reasons to pursue solutions.

This chapter describes a structured teamwork system that is being
tested and used in emergency departments around the country to
reduce the risk of clinical errors. Small teams of caregivers with different sets of clinical skills are learning to work closely and in a coordinated fashion to define, execute, and monitor the delivery of care to
patients assigned to the team. The goal of such teamwork is to provide
the highest standard of care to all patients belonging to the team.

Patients in other acute care units of the hospital are also likely to
benefit significantly from this type of teamwork system. The application
of this structured teamwork approach could possibly reduce clinical
errors in other high-stress/high-performance environments where caregivers are often forced to deliver care to patients under conditions of
incomplete information. These units include the following:

- Labor and delivery units
- Special care units (intensive care, critical care, neonatal inten-
  sive care, and so on)
- Operating rooms
- Postanesthesia care units
- Emergency medical services teams

Caregivers in these units are often forced to manage care delivery
to several unstable patients simultaneously. Communication conditions are often less than ideal, and patients can face grave and immediate consequences if mistreatment occurs. The stresses on caregivers
for high standards of performance are great. Tight coordination is
essential and caregivers must respond quickly to changing situations. It
seems likely that the MedTeams teamwork system could help in each
of these environments.

Readers will also be introduced to one of the tools of the teamwork
system, the Teamwork Failure Checklist. This checklist can be used by
caregivers during an incident or accident investigation to identify teamwork failures that contributed to the event. This tool, originally
designed by Dynamics Research Corporation for an analysis of ED
closed claims, can help organizations recognize the teamwork breakdowns that contributed to the undesirable patient care event. The

checklist can also be used prospectively to identify and correct inadequate teamwork performance that could lead to a sentinel event.

TEAMWORK CHALLENGES IN EMERGENCY CARE

Although individual clinical errors can, and sometimes do, precipitate dramatic adverse events, it is often a sequence of errors (an "error chain") that precipitates such events.[33,34] The only positive aspect to such error chains is that they commonly unfold over a period of time and consequently provide significant opportunities for caregivers to recognize the emerging problem and intervene to break the chain. The following is a summary of an actual closed malpractice case where the chain was never broken. This case reveals several common teamwork failures and demonstrates the potentially dramatic consequences.

A female in her late thirties came to the emergency department reporting an increased incidence of her normal angina chest pains over the preceding two weeks. She denied any current chest pain when the triage nurse inquired, but did report some mild shortness of breath. The patient had a long history of heart disease, including documented coronary artery disease. She was on multiple medications. She was triaged as "urgent," the second highest triage category in a four-tier triage system, even though she had abnormal vital signs and a significant history that should have placed her in the highest category, "emergent patient." The ED was extremely busy and the patient was in the department for almost one hour before being evaluated by a medical student. The patient complained of mild (3 on a scale of 1 to 10) chest pain and was found to have virtually no pulse in her limbs. One-and-a-half hours after presentation to the ED, repeat vital signs by the nurse showed very low blood pressure (61/32). This was not communicated to the medical student or the physician. To relieve the patient's chest pain, the physician ordered nitroglycerin (NTG) to be given under the tongue. During the investigation following this incident, the nurse reported on a written statement that she was uncomfortable giving NTG, a drug that will lower blood pressure, to a patient with very low blood pressure (hypotension); however, she indicated that she thought the physician "knew what he was doing."

The patient continued to complain of chest pain and shortness of breath so another drug (morphine sulfate) and an NTG intravenous drip were instituted. Almost one-half hour after the initial hypotensive episode, the patient's low blood pressure was noted by the physician and the NTG infusion was discontinued. At this time a consult with the internal medicine resident was called, and the resident arrived in the ED one-half hour later. The patient remained hypotensive, and her chest pain and extreme breathing difficulties (dyspnea) worsened. The patient became extremely hypotensive, her heart rate dropped far below normal, and the "code team" was activated. Cardiac resuscitation, including epinephrine, atropine, defibrillation, external pacing, and pericardiocentesis, was unsuccessful. The patient was pronounced dead three hours and ten minutes after entering the ED.[35]

This case demonstrates a chain of errors in which poor climate, lack of team structure, poor task priority setting, poor communication, and lack of cross-monitoring and assertiveness within the ED contributed to a catastrophic patient outcome that sadly rippled into the lives of many people. The consequences of this team failure were dramatic: the patient died, the family was devastated, the staff was distressed and demoralized, the hospital's reputation was harmed, and over $2 million was paid in settlement.[36]

Teamwork failures like these are more common than most clinicians or patients want to believe. For example, Dynamics Research Corporation found in a 1997 retrospective review of ED closed claims arising from 4.7 million patient visits, that consequential teamwork failures occurred in 43 percent of the ED closed claims.[37,38] For this 43 percent, the average number of teamwork failures per case was 8.8 (ranging from 1 to 32). The teamwork failures most frequently cited in the study as contributing to clinical errors are shown in figure 9-1. Note that the single teamwork failure most frequently cited as contributing to the occurrence of clinical error was "cross-monitoring." A cross-monitoring failure refers to a failure to recognize a clinical error created by one caregiver that was readily visible and could have been caught by another caregiver. Such failures occur all too frequently in

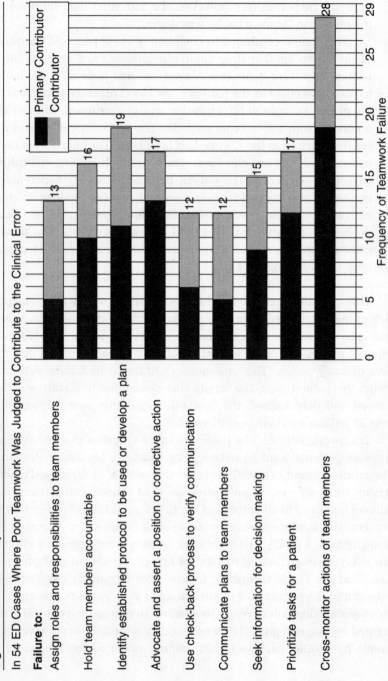

Figure 9-1. Most Frequent Teamwork Errors

In 54 ED Cases Where Poor Teamwork Was Judged to Contribute to the Clinical Error

Failure to:

- Assign roles and responsibilities to team members — 13
- Hold team members accountable — 16
- Identify established protocol to be used or develop a plan — 19
- Advocate and assert a position or corrective action — 17
- Use check-back process to verify communication — 12
- Communicate plans to team members — 12
- Seek information for decision making — 15
- Prioritize tasks for a patient — 17
- Cross-monitor actions of team members — 28

Frequency of Teamwork Failure

Primary Contributor
Contributor

the current culture because it is generally unacceptable behavior for one caregiver to check another caregiver's actions. The care community has done little to cultivate such monitoring habits and much to inhibit them.

Perhaps the most alarming fact was that eight of the twelve deaths reviewed were judged to be preventable if appropriate teamwork action had been taken. Moreover, five of the eight major permanent impairments (for example, significant heart damage, loss of a limb, loss of ability to manage daily living activities) were judged to be preventable if appropriate teamwork actions had been taken.

In addition, it was estimated that better ED teamwork, on average, would save $560,479 per closed case where teamwork can influence the outcome (that is, prevent or mitigate the error). Examined from another perspective, this turns out to be $345,460 in savings per 100,000 ED patients, or nearly $3.50 for every patient seen by the ED. This is believed to be a conservative estimate of true costs that could be avoided by better teamwork.[39,40]

THE TEAMWORK SYSTEM

The summary presented here is an overview of the teamwork system created by the MedTeams Project, a large applied research project that has developed an emergency care teamwork system that has been implemented at 10 hospitals across the country.[41] This teamwork system is designed to improve care delivery performance and reduce the occurrence of clinical errors. It teaches team members to actively coordinate and support each other in the course of clinical task execution using the structure of work teams. Teams and teamwork behaviors do not replace clinical skills but rather serve to ensure that clinical activities are properly integrated and executed to deliver effective emergency care. Teamwork is a management tool to expedite care delivery to patients, a mechanism to give caregivers increased control over their constantly changing environment, and a safety net to help protect both patients and caregivers from inevitable human failings and their consequences. The basic concepts and behaviors of teamwork are taught to staff in a one-day course. The behaviors taught become habits and skills through daily practice.

Team Definition and Composition

Early on in the MedTeams Project it was found that ED caregivers often had an expanded, varied, and abstract concept of a "team" that lacked the precision necessary to create practical, manageable work teams. They tended to include within the team boundary not only the many members of the ED staff but also members of other departments, such as laboratory, housekeeping, and administration. This was "team" in the big-group, loose sense of the word. For the teamwork system to be effective, a tighter, narrower definition of "team" had to be introduced. The ED needed to create small, mission-focused, technically skilled teams similar to those of the cockpit crews in aviation.

In the MedTeams System an ED core team consists of a set of three to as many as ten clinically skilled caregivers who have been trained to use specific teamwork behavior to tightly coordinate and manage their clinical actions. (Average core team size in the project was six.) Each core team contains at least one physician and one nurse. The most experienced physician on the team is usually the team leader. The team leader only serves as leader to one team during a specific work shift. Team members always know who is on their team and who is the team leader. To make coordination easier, individuals who are members of the same team commonly wear a unique, readily visible identifier (such as a colored patch, an armband or badge, a type or color of clothing, and so on) that denotes an individual as belonging to a specific team.

Team Responsibilities

The goal of each ED core team is to deliver high-quality ED clinical care to the set of ED patients assigned to it. To achieve this goal, team members coordinate directly and repeatedly with each other to ensure proper and timely clinical task execution and to detect and help overloaded teammates. Each team member works to maintain a clear understanding (a common situation awareness) of the care status and care plan for each patient assigned to the team and the workload status of each team member. Teams hold brief meetings to make team decisions, assign/reassign responsibilities and tasks, establish/reestablish situation awareness, and learn lessons.

The team oversees and directly manages the use of all care resources needed by the patients assigned to the team. Figure 9-2 shows

Figure 9-2. Care Resources Managed by the ED Core Team

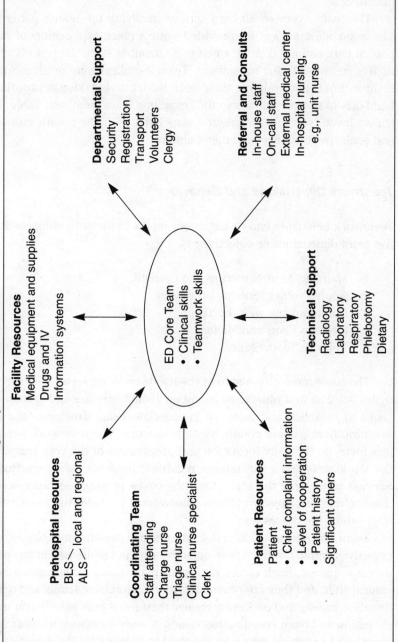

Facility Resources
Medical equipment and supplies
Drugs and IV
Information systems

Prehospital resources
BLS ⟩ local and regional
ALS ⟩

Coordinating Team
Staff attending
Charge nurse
Triage nurse
Clinical nurse specialist
Clerk

ED Core Team
• Clinical skills
• Teamwork skills

Departmental Support
Security
Registration
Transport
Volunteers
Clergy

Referral and Consults
In-house staff
On-call staff
External medical center
In-hospital nursing,
e.g., unit nurse

Technical Support
Radiology
Laboratory
Respiratory
Phlebotomy
Dietary

Patient Resources
Patient
• Chief complaint information
• Level of cooperation
• Patient history
Significant others

the range of care resources commonly used by the team to support patient care.

The team oversees all care actions involving the team's patients. The team must always be provided with a clear explanation of any patient care action taken by a non-team-member since the team is ultimately responsible for the patient. Team members may not leave the team without first notifying their team leader and making appropriate hand-offs of responsibilities to the remaining team members. Table 9-1 shows basic team characteristics associated with the team's mission and goals, performance, and membership.

Teamwork Dimensions and Behaviors

Teamwork behaviors can be organized into a framework composed of five team dimensions or objectives:

1. Maintain Team Structure and Climate.
2. Apply Problem-Solving Strategies.
3. Communicate with the Team.
4. Execute Plans and Manage Workloads.
5. Improve Team Skills.

The basic interrelationship of the five team dimensions is shown in figure 9-3. The first objective—Maintain Team Structure and Climate—seeks to establish and maintain appropriate team structures and an organizational climate conducive to teamwork. The teamwork behaviors focus on the daily formation and preparation of the core team for the work shift and expectations regarding professional interactions. Success in meeting the other four objectives presupposes success in meeting this first objective; Team Dimension 1 provides the foundation upon which the others rest.

Team Dimensions 2, 3, and 4 address daily operational teamwork objectives within the ED. These objectives are not addressed in any particular sequence. Each comes into focus many times in the course of a clinical shift, and they are often intertwined. Moreover, teams and team members rapidly and frequently change their focus between clinical task execution and team coordination issues. A team member's focus at any given point in time is driven by the need to balance (1) the demands of the immediate patient care requirements against (2) the need to monitor

Table 9-1.   Team Characteristics

Factor	Characteristics
Mission and goals	• Teams are oriented to accomplishing a well-defined, time-bound objective. • There is a definable standard of performance.
Performance	• Teams have a time orientation to their work. The team has an identifiable start and stop time for its tasks and duties. • There is real-time communication by team members. • Members operate in parallel and their actions must be coordinated. • Certain team tasks are routine and can be choreographed or scripted. Other aspects of working together are ad hoc coordination and can only be guided by teamwork rules and principles. • Decision making takes place (planned or on-the-fly) that immediately affects the team's care delivery actions. • Members coordinate to develop and execute plans. • Teams actively intervene to eliminate task overloads on individual team members whenever possible. • A team can improve its performance through practice and after-action review.
Membership	• Individuals can identify themselves as members of the team. • Team membership is structured. The roles of leader and follower are understood by the team members, but there are opportunities for emergent leadership and followership roles depending on the demands of patient care and the skills of the team member. • Team membership is driven by the skill mix the team mission requires. Partial overlap of skills permits a degree of flexibility in task assignment within the team. • During the temporal life of the team, the team's duties are superordinate to the personal goals of the individual team members.

Figure 9-3.   The Interrelationships of the Five Team Dimensions

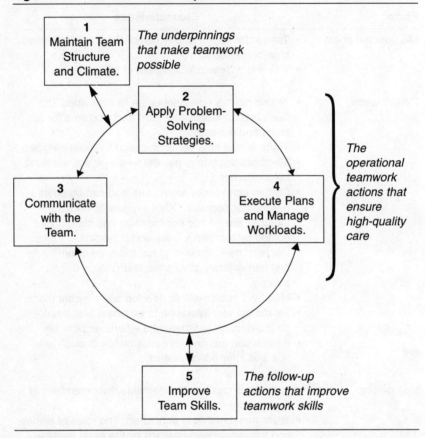

and maintain situation awareness in order to prevent errors and ensure the quality of impending care.

Team Dimension 2—Apply Problem-Solving Strategies—brings caregivers face to face with their human fallibility as it relates to the decision-making process and judgment biases. This objective addresses actions that can be taken to minimize the occurrence of errors within the team. Success in applying many of the error-avoidance actions identified in this dimension is dependent on team members holding a common understanding of the care plan and the status of care plan execution for each patient.

Team Dimension 3—Communicate with the Team—focuses on communication activities that help team members establish and maintain a common understanding of patient and operational issues affecting team and teammate workload levels. This objective is generally focused on timely and accurate information transfer and on maintaining a common situation awareness so team members can effectively coordinate actions and recognize pending errors. By "situation awareness" we mean one's level of awareness of important mission-related information and events that are occurring in the immediate operational environment.[42] In the emergency care world this means an awareness of the patient status and care plan for patients assigned to the team and awareness of the workload levels of fellow team members. This dimension addresses specific teamwork actions taken to ensure timely and accurate clinical communication. Team members cannot deliver proper care or effectively coordinate actions without an accurate awareness of the current state of affairs.

The fourth team objective or dimension—Execute Plans and Manage Workloads—focuses on eliminating immediate work overload on individual team members by having team members help each other with tasks. Task assistance is a risk-avoidance activity that reduces the potential for clinical errors that stem from stress, fatigue, lack of the necessary skills, or individual overload. The concept is simple—help others and ask for help.

The last teamwork objective—Improve Team Skills—focuses on improving teamwork skills through team review meetings, one-on-one coaching, and situation-specific teaching conducted during real-time patient care activities. In this dimension, shift reviews enable the team to examine the experiences during the shift, discuss the teamwork and care performance, and provide immediate lessons and feedback to team members. The coaching and teaching actions provide similar insights and feedback. This dimension is important because it provides a feedback mechanism to revise and improve the team's performance. Establishing new habits and skills requires regular practice. Absorbing new concepts takes time.

Primary descriptors for each team dimension or objective are found in table 9-2, the Teamwork Behavior Matrix. Primary descriptors help organize course training materials. The practical daily actions actually taken by team members for each team dimension are found in the last column in the matrix.

Team Activities

There are two basic categories of teamwork activity: teamwork conferences and individual teamwork. Teamwork conferences refer to those

Table 9-2. Teamwork Behavior Matrix

TD#	Team Dimension	Primary Descriptors	Teamwork Actions by Core Team
1	Maintain team structure and climate.	Establish leadership.	a) Establish the leader.
		Organize team.	b) Assemble the team.
			c) Assign roles and responsibilities.
			d) Communicate essential team information.
		Cultivate team climate.	e) Acknowledge the contributions of team members to team goals.
			f) Demonstrate mutual respect in all communications.
			g) Hold each other accountable for team outcomes.
		Resolve conflicts.	h) Address professional concerns directly.
			i) Resolve conflicts constructively.
2	Apply problem-solving strategies.	Conduct situational planning.	a) Engage team members in planning process.
			b) Identify established protocol to be used or develop a plan.
		Apply decision-making methods.	c) Engage team members in decision-making process.
		Engage in error-correction actions.	d) Alert team to potential biases and errors.
			e) Report slips, lapses, and mistakes to team.
			f) Advocate and assert a position or corrective action.
			g) Invoke the Two-Challenge Rule when an initial assertion is ignored.
3	Communicate with the team.	Maintain situational awareness.	a) Request situation awareness updates.
			b) Provide situation awareness updates.
		Use standards of communication.	c) Use ED common terminology in all communications.
			d) Call out critical information during emergent events.

e) Use check-backs to verify information transfer.
f) Systematically hand off responsibilities during team transitions.

Offer information to team.

g) Offer information to support planning and decision making.
h) Communicate decisions and actions to team members.

Request information from team.

i) Seek information for planning and decision making.

4 Execute plans and manage workload.

Implement plan.

a) Execute protocol or team-established plan.
b) Integrate individual assessments of patient needs.

Conduct secondary triage.

c) Re-plan patient care in response to overall caseload of team.

Prioritize tasks.

d) Prioritize tasks for individual patients.

Cross-monitor.

e) Cross-monitor actions of team members.

Manage team resources and workload.

f) Balance workload within the team.
g) Request assistance for task overload.
h) Offer assistance for task overload.
i) Constructively use periods of low workload.

5 Improve team skills.

Engage in informal team improvement strategies.

a) Engage in situational learning and teaching with the team.
b) Engage in coaching with team members.
c) Conduct shift reviews of teamwork.
d) Conduct event reviews of teamwork.

Engage in formal team improvement strategies.

e) Participate in educational forums addressing teamwork.
f) Participate in clinical case reviews examining teamwork.

few times during the shift when the full team comes together for a meeting. There are usually only a few of these meetings each shift unless the team is very small (two or three caregivers) because it is simply too difficult to convene the full group. Most commonly there is one meeting at the beginning of the shift and one near the end of the shift.[43] Each meeting typically lasts two to three minutes. These meetings are most often used to assign duties, establish situation awareness, gather information, discuss problems, or learn lessons.

The bulk of the teamwork activities are done by caregivers operating as individual team members observing or briefly connecting with one other team member. Common individual team members' teamwork actions could include the following:

- Caregiver A helps B with a clinical task. (A and B could be any two members of the team.)
- Caregiver A observes B's actions and notes nothing unusual so no direct interaction occurs.
- Caregiver A corrects B's situation awareness when she notes an unexpected care action by B.
- Caregiver A alerts B to the fact that he is about to make an error so B alters his action.
- Caregiver A informs B that he has made an error and they initiate corrective actions.
- Caregiver A discovers an error by B, initiates corrective actions, and alerts B and the team to the error and the actions taken.
- Caregiver A has her own situation awareness corrected by B when she asks a question about a presumed error.

These are examples of actions that give teamwork its operational power. Teamwork at the operational level involves an integration of these actions into a recurring intermittent process of monitoring, intervening, and correcting errors or deviations in situation awareness. These actions are known as "check" actions. Such actions are just another part of the common daily work activities of team members. Each team member readily moves between clinical tasks and check tasks as a part of the normal process of caring for patients and monitoring for errors. A model of the basic teamwork check cycle employed by caregivers is shown in figure 9-4.[44]

The teamwork check cycle begins with each team member monitoring his or her own situation awareness (1) and cross-monitoring

Figure 9-4. The Teamwork Check Cycle

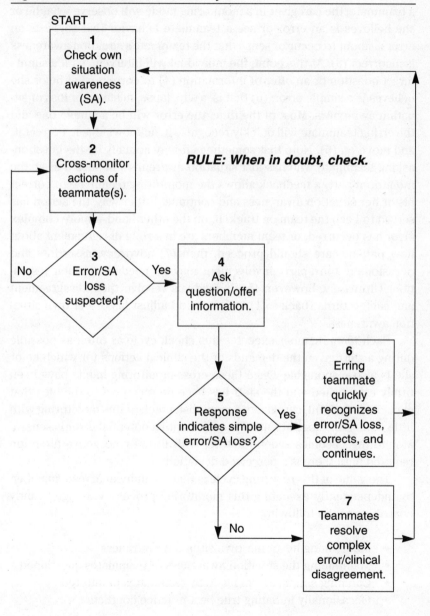

(2) the actions of his or her teammates. Occasionally when monitoring a teammate, the caregiver in a monitoring mode will observe what he or she believes is an error or see a teammate behavior that suggests an error is about to occur or sense that the teammate's situation awareness is incorrect (3). At this point, the individual will intervene with a simple direct question or an offer of information (4) to correct what he or she believes is a simple error; (5) that is, a slip, lapse, mistake, or loss of situation awareness. Most of the time, the error will be a simple one and the erring teammate will quickly recognize it, acknowledge it, correct it, and move on (6). Note that sometimes it may actually be the question-asking teammate who has lost situation awareness. In such a case, the monitored party's feedback allows the monitoring teammate to correct his or her situation awareness and continue. Either way, the action has served to keep the team on track. If, on the other hand, a more complex error has occurred, or team members are in strong disagreement about how patient care should proceed, then (7) advocacy, assertion, and occasionally third-party involvement may be needed to reach resolution. Ultimately, however, the individuals resolve their disagreement and each returns (back to 1) to check and adjust his or her own situation awareness.

Each team member executes this check cycle as often as possible during a shift given the demands of the clinical actions for which he or she is also responsible. Once these cross-monitoring habits have been firmly established and the staff has become receptive to the idea that checking is helpful, caregivers accomplish much of this monitoring with little or no conscious attention required until a potential error is sensed. Monitoring becomes second nature, with little or no active attention required until there is a perceived deviation.

The value of this recurring cycle is that the individual team member, by independently executing this monitoring process, can significantly contribute to the following:

- Maintaining his or her own situation awareness
- Maintaining the situation awareness of teammates questioned
- Catching simple errors made by teammates monitored
- Occasionally initiating true best-practice conflicts

Note that although in reality there are few actual conflicts in teams over what is the best practice for a particular patient, it is extremely important for the effective functioning of the teamwork system that staff know they will not have their "heads cut off" for challenging an action that they believe may harm the patient. Doctors and nurses in this teamwork system learn to explain their actions in a calm, civil manner. This openness is imperative because if the senior members of the team intimidate the junior members with sharp rebukes, the junior members will not be willing to inquire about apparently simple errors for fear that they will inadvertently stumble into best-practice disagreements. If open communication is suppressed, simple slips and lapses will not get caught.

Over time the recurring monitoring actions of the check cycle become part of the ingrained habits of each caregiver. The aggregate impact of multiple team members simultaneously and continuously conducting the check cycle as a normal part of their daily work routine is dramatic: hundreds of checks on the team each day. Conscientious use of the teamwork check cycle breaks error chains. (Additional details on the MedTeams Teamwork System are available at Web site http://teams.drc.com.)

IDENTIFYING TEAMWORK FAILURES IN INCIDENTS

There is a growing recognition in the health care world that organizations must learn from the incidents that occur. The Joint Commission for Accreditation of Healthcare Organizations has made this recognition explicit in its new sentinel event guidance.[45] In addition, individual hospitals and facilities are beginning to recognize the need to learn about their system weaknesses from less dramatic incidents that are also symptoms of system failure. The teamwork failure checklist (figure 9-5) is a tool to help organizations gain insight into system weaknesses as they relate to teamwork. It allows the organization to identify teamwork failures that contributed to the error. The insight gained from the assessment permits the organization to consider teamwork improvement options (for example, revise work structures to establish teams, provide staff training in teamwork, or alter reward structures) and make appropriate plans for system improvement. And where a sentinel event has occurred, the checklist can provide an assessment of teamwork breakdowns and aid in determining if they contributed to the error occurrence. Completion of the checklist becomes a component of the formal root cause analysis (RCA).

Figure 9-5.   Teamwork Failure Checklist

Case or Claim Code # _____

Reviewer Codes _____

Description of Error/Incident _____

(Describe the error in a short, brief sentence.)

PART A—Assessment of Teamwork Failures That Contributed to the Error

Instructions: Thoroughly review the available facts of the case before beginning. For each teamwork behavior answer each question by marking "Yes" or "No" with an X. Answer each of the four assessment questions in order from left to right until you make a "No" response or complete question 4. Then move to question 1 for the next teamwork behavior and repeat the assessment process. Continue until all the teamwork behaviors have been reviewed.

TD Code	Teamwork Behavior	1. Was the behavior appropriate for the situation?		2. Was there a teamwork behavior failure?		3. Did the failure contribute to the error?		4. Was the failure a primary contributor to the error?	
		No	Yes	No	Yes	No	Yes	No	Yes
1	a) Establish the leader		X→		→		→		
	b) Assemble the team		X→		→		→		
	c) Assign roles and responsibilities		X→		→		→		
	d) Communicate essential team information		X→		→		→		
	e) Acknowledge the contributions of team members to team goals		→		→		→		
	f) Demonstrate mutual respect in all communication		X→		→		→		
	g) Hold each other accountable for team outcomes		X→		→		→		
	h) Address professional concerns directly		→		→		→		
	i) Resolve conflicts constructively		→		→		→		
2	a) Engage team members in planning process		X→		→		→		
	b) Identify established protocol to be used or develop a plan		X→		→		→		
	c) Engage team members in decision-making process		→		→		→		
	d) Alert team to potential biases and errors		→		→		→		

Figure 9-5.   (Continued)

TD Code	Teamwork Behavior	1. Was the behavior appropriate for the situation?		2. Was there a teamwork behavior failure?		3. Did the failure contribute to the error?		4. Was the failure a primary contributor to the error?	
		No	Yes	No	Yes	No	Yes	No	Yes
	e) Report slips, lapses, and mistakes to team		→		→		→		
	f) Advocate and assert a position or corrective action		→		→		→		
	g) Invoke the Two-Challenge Rule when an initial assertion is ignored		→		→		→		
3	a) Request situation awareness updates	X→			→		→		
	b) Provide situation awareness updates	X→			→		→		
	c) Use ED common terminology in all communications	X→			→		→		
	d) Call out critical information during emergent events		→		→		→		
	e) Use check-backs to verify information transfer	X→			→		→		
	f) Systematically hand off responsibilities during team transitions	X→			→		→		
	g) Offer information to support planning and decision making		→		→		→		
	h) Communicate decisions and actions to team members	X→			→		→		
	i) Seek information for planning and decision making		→		→		→		
4	a) Execute protocol or team-established plan	X→			→		→		
	b) Integrate individual assessments of patient needs		→		→		→		
	c) Re-plan patient care in response to overall caseload of team	X→			→		→		
	d) Prioritize tasks for individual patients	X→			→		→		
	e) Cross-monitor actions of team members	X→			→		→		
	f) Balance workload within the team	X→			→		→		

(Continued on next page)

Figure 9-5. (Continued)

TD Code	Teamwork Behavior	1. Was the behavior appropriate for the situation?		2. Was there a teamwork behavior failure?		3. Did the failure contribute to the error?		4. Was the failure a primary contributor to the error?	
		No	Yes	No	Yes	No	Yes	No	Yes
	g) Request assistance for task overload		→		→		→		
	h) Offer assistance for task overload		→		→		→		
	i) Constructively use periods of low workload		→		→		→		
5	a) Engage in situational learning and teaching with the team		→		→		→		
	b) Engage in coaching with team members		→		→		→		
	c) Conduct shift reviews of teamwork	X→			→		→		
	d) Conduct event reviews of teamwork		→		→		→		
	e) Participate in educational forums addressing teamwork		→		→		→		
	f) Participate in clinical case reviews examining teamwork		→		→		→		

PART B
Assessing the Impact of Effective Teamwork

Question 3. What impact would effective teamwork have had on this case? (Circle one answer.)

a.) Would <u>have prevented</u> the error(s) from occurring.

b.) Would <u>have mitigated</u> the impact of the error(s) but not have prevented it.

c.) Would <u>not have prevented</u> the error(s) or mitigated the impact of the error(s).

Completion of the Checklist

For any one incident, the completion of the teamwork failure checklist is a three-stage process (figure 9-6): (1) collect the facts, (2) review the facts, and (3) complete the checklist. The main objective in the fact collection phase is to bring all the facts together into one file so that the data can be easily reviewed. When the incident has been brought to the attention of the risk manager shortly after its occurrence and the risk manager has initiated a claim file to capture the relevant facts, significant amounts of reliable data will be available. If a claim file is not initiated until a suit is filed (often months or years after the incident), the quality and completeness of the data will be dramatically reduced, making completion of the teamwork failure checklist difficult, if not impossible.

Unless the parties conducting the formal interviews of the caregivers involved in the incident specifically ask questions regarding the interactions between the caregivers, interview reports typically are silent

Figure 9-6.   Individual Claim Assessment Process

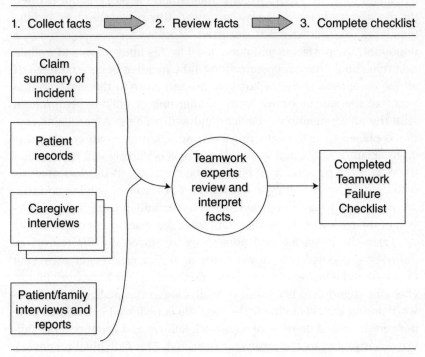

on the coordination actions between caregivers. Caregiver coordination information was often missing in the retrospective review of incidents conducted by Dynamics Research Corporation. If you intend to evaluate team performance in future incidents, it is strongly recommended that you ask the risk manager to ensure that all future caregiver interviews include detailed questions about the communication and coordination actions. Direct questions about these actions provide the best facts and insights for assessing teamwork. However, recognize that where no claim file exists it will be very difficult, and in many cases impossible, to acquire the incident data after the fact.

In the second phase of completing the checklist, the collected facts are reviewed and interpreted to understand the incident story. This interpretation is most effectively accomplished by using a physician-nurse pair (p-n pair), in particular a pair who are seasoned caregivers and have had formal training in teamwork. It is better still if they have had experience working in a team-based emergency care system or another team-structured unit. The pairing is needed because physicians and nurses often have very different views of the world. Both perspectives tend to be necessary to fully understand the story, and it is often the discussions between the two reviewers that reveal the story and the teamwork breakdowns that occurred. Moreover, since objectivity is important, the physician and nurse used in this integration and evaluation role should have no connection to the incident being examined. If all the caregivers in the department are too close to the incident, it is best that the pair be drawn from another unit or outside organization with the above-mentioned background and training. A particular caution is placed against conducting a review and interpretation using only a physician or only a nurse; the risk of bias occurring will be high and the risk of the perception of bias will be even higher. Incident analysis by a lone reviewer will raise questions of assessment validity and trigger resistance to any proposed solutions stemming from it. The selection of the reviewers is an important issue for assessment credibility.

Once the physician and nurse have reviewed the file (caregiver interviews, depositions, patient records, and/or case summaries) and understand the incident chronology and the story, the teamwork failure checklist (figure 9-5) is used to formally assess the quality of the teamwork during the event chain. The case file is reviewed in detail and the p-n pair decides if there were teamwork failures and whether those failures contributed to the error that occurred. The individual teamwork behaviors, shown in column two of the checklist, are grouped according to the relevant team dimensions (see column 2 of the matrix in table 9-2). Each teamwork behavior shown in the checklist is assessed by answering a sequence of four contingent questions:

1. Was the behavior appropriate for the situation?
2. Was there a teamwork behavior failure?
3. Did the failure contribute to the error?
4. Was the failure a primary contributor to the error?

For each teamwork behavior the two reviewers move horizontally through the series of four questions shown in columns 3 through 6 on the checklist. Question-asking continues until either one of the four questions is answered "no" or all four questions have been answered. The reviewers then move to the next teamwork behavior and repeat the four-question sequence. This process is repeated until all teamwork behaviors have been reviewed.

The teamwork failure checklist comes preprinted with an "X" in the "yes" column for the first question for some teamwork behaviors. These teamwork behaviors are considered to be applicable for all situations. For example, the teamwork behavior "Establish the leader" (1a) is always an applicable behavior. The team should never be in doubt regarding who is the leader. If any one of the caregivers involved in the incident indicates in an interview that he was uncertain who was the leader, then there was a teamwork failure with respect to this behavior and an "X" would be placed in the "yes" column for question 2. And, continuing with this example, if the caregiver's focus on trying to discover who was the leader contributed to his forgetting to give a medication to a patient and that patient later went into convulsions because he had not received the needed drug, then the teamwork failure would be a contributor to the incident. In this instance, an "X" would be placed in the "yes" column for question 3. The failure to designate a leader could even become a primary contributor (question 4) if a conflict erupted between two caregivers over who was leader during a code and the conflict delayed delivery of time-critical care and the patient died. Recognize that the judgment of the extent to which the teamwork failure contributed to the clinical error occurrence requires an understanding of the clinical situation, the clinical options available, and the teamwork actions possible.

Note that there are also teamwork behaviors where the first question has not been pre-answered with a "yes" in the first question. These teamwork behaviors are only appropriate under particular situations. For example, if the staff were under conditions of high workload during the incident and the entire shift, then obviously the teamwork behavior "constructively use periods of low workload" (4i) is not relevant to the situation surrounding the incident. Similarly, if there is neither perceived nor real caregiver disagreement in an incident, then "Advocate and assert a position or corrective action" (2f) is not a relevant teamwork behavior given the case situation. One would not expect a caregiver to display this behavior. "Advocating a position" would be nonsense behavior in the absence of a perceived or real disagreement.

The last question on the form (after the individual behaviors have all been reviewed) asks the p-n pair to decide what impact they believe sound teamwork would have had on the error associated with the incident. It asks the pair to decide if proper teamwork would have prevented the error, mitigated the impact of the error, or had no impact on the error. To answer this question the pair should first review the checklist and the decisions they made regarding the individual teamwork behaviors and then decide whether they believe better teamwork could have prevented or mitigated the error. The pair might also wish to prepare a summary statement explaining their position on the impact of the teamwork failures on the clinical error.

Figure 9-7 shows a completed teamwork failure checklist for the analysis that was conducted for the earlier described incident involving the young woman presenting with chest pain who died as a result of poor care. This incident occurred in an ED environment with no formal team structure and a poor organizational climate. During the woman's stay in the ED there were multiple caregiver communication failures and there was a dramatic lack of caregiver assertiveness on behalf of the patient. The patient should have been triaged as "emergent" at arrival and should have immediately received medical attention and a thorough workup. Cross-monitoring by any caregiver with even basic clinical training should have surfaced this triage error and the high risk involved in giving nitroglycerin to a patient with low blood pressure. None of the needed teamwork actions that could have broken this error chain occurred.

Several of the team behaviors are checked as "not appropriate" in this situation. These behaviors involve teaching and coaching and work

Figure 9-7. Example of Completed Teamwork Failure Checklist

Case or Claim Code # _____2372_____

Reviewer Codes _____Dr. J & Nurse Z_____

Description of Error/Incident _Failure to recognize and treat hypotensive crisis._

(Describe the error in a short, brief sentence.)

PART A—Assessment of Teamwork Failures That Contributed to the Error

Instructions: Thoroughly review the available facts of the case before beginning. For each teamwork behavior answer each question by marking "Yes" or "No" with an X. Answer each of the four assessment questions in order from left to right until you make a "No" response or complete question 4. Then move to question 1 for the next teamwork behavior and repeat the assessment process. Continue until all the teamwork behaviors have been reviewed. *(Note that for this example we used a √ (check) to show the evaluator entry more clearly.)*

TD Code	Teamwork Behavior	1. Was the behavior appropriate for the situation?		2. Was there a teamwork behavior failure?		3. Did the failure contribute to the error?		4. Was the failure a primary contributor to the error?	
		No	Yes	No	Yes	No	Yes	No	Yes
1	a) Establish the leader		X→		√→		√→		√
	b) Assemble the team		X→		√→		√→	√	
	c) Assign roles and responsibilities		X→	√	→		→		→
	d) Communicate essential team information		X→	√	→		→		→
	e) Acknowledge the contributions of team members to team goals	√	→		→		→		→
	f) Demonstrate mutual respect in all communication		X→	√	→		→		→
	g) Hold each other accountable for team outcomes		X→		√→		√→	√	
	h) Address professional concerns directly		√→		√→		√→		√
	i) Resolve conflicts constructively		√→		√→		√→	√	
2	a) Engage team members in planning process		X→		√→		√→	√	
	b) Identify established protocol to be used or develop a plan		X→		√→		√→		√
	c) Engage team members in decision-making process		√→		√→		√→	√	
	d) Alert team to potential biases and errors		√→		√→		√→	√	

(Continued on next page)

Figure 9-7. (Continued)

TD Code	Teamwork Behavior	1. Was the behavior appropriate for the situation?		2. Was there a teamwork behavior failure?		3. Did the failure contribute to the error?		4. Was the failure a primary contributor to the error?	
		No	Yes	No	Yes	No	Yes	No	Yes
	e) Report slips, lapses, and mistakes to team		√→	√→		√→		√	
	f) Advocate and assert a position or corrective action		√→	√→		√→			√
	g) Invoke the Two-Challenge Rule when an initial assertion is ignored	√	→		→		→		
3	a) Request situation awareness updates		X→	√→		√→		√	
	b) Provide situation awareness updates		X→	√→		√→		√	
	c) Use ED common terminology in all communications		X→	√	→		→		
	d) Call out critical information during emergent events	√	→		→		→		
	e) Use check-backs to verify information transfer		X→	√	→		→		
	f) Systematically hand off responsibilities during team transitions		X→	√	→		→		
	g) Offer information to support planning and decision making		√→	√→		√→			√
	h) Communicate decisions and actions to team members		X→	√→		√→		√	
	i) Seek information for planning and decision making		√→	√→		√→			√
4	a) Execute protocol or team-established plan		X→	√	→		→		
	b) Integrate individual assessments of patient needs		√→	√→		√→		√	
	c) Re-plan patient care in response to overall caseload of team		X→	√	→		→		
	d) Prioritize tasks for individual patients		X→	√→		√→		√	
	e) Cross-monitor actions of team members		X→	√→		√→			√
	f) Balance workload within the team		X→	√	→		→		

Figure 9-7. (Continued)

TD Code	Teamwork Behavior	1. Was the behavior appropriate for the situation?		2. Was there a teamwork behavior failure?		3. Did the failure contribute to the error?		4. Was the failure a primary contributor to the error?	
		No	Yes	No	Yes	No	Yes	No	Yes
	g) Request assistance for task overload	√	→		→		→		
	h) Offer assistance for task overload	√	→		→		→		
	i) Constructively use periods of low workload	√	→		→		→		
5	a) Engage in situational learning and teaching with the team	√	→		→		→		
	b) Engage in coaching with team members	√	→		→		→		
	c) Conduct shift reviews of teamwork	X→	√		→		→		
	d) Conduct event reviews of teamwork		√→	√→		√	→		
	e) Participate in educational forums addressing teamwork	√	→		→		→		
	f) Participate in clinical case reviews examining teamwork	√	→		→		→		

PART B
Assessing the Impact of Effective Teamwork

Question 3. What impact would effective teamwork have had on this case?
(Circle one answer.)

a.) Would <u>have prevented</u> the error(s) from occurring.

b.) Would <u>have mitigated</u> the impact of the error(s) but not have prevented it.

c.) Would <u>not have prevented</u> the error(s) or mitigated the impact of the error(s).

environment. It was determined by the p-n pair reviewing this event that while the ED was busy at the time the woman presented, this was not a situation of task overload triggering the errors. Poor organizational climate appears to have been the chief culprit because it significantly undermined communication among caregivers. Both the climate and the busy pace of the ED probably precluded real-time situation teaching and coaching and may have sabotaged opportunities for team reviews during the shift.

Furthermore, note that team reviews and case reviews/forums addressing teamwork concerns almost never help break the error chain while an event is still unfolding. These education actions more commonly have a delayed impact; that is, they make the caregivers smarter and more capable of recognizing and breaking error chains in future incidents. Only when an error chain unfolds very slowly over a period of many hours or perhaps days can team reviews and case reviews/forums possibly contribute to the breaking of a specific unfolding chain. In general, Team Dimension 5 actions are not primary contributors to the breaking of error chains.

As shown in part B of the teamwork failure checklist, the p-n pair reviewing the incident felt that effective teamwork *would* have prevented the error from occurring. In the 1997 retrospective analysis of ED closed claims, Dynamics Research Corporation found that the participating p-n pairs generally thought that in cases with two or more "primary contributor" teamwork failures, proper teamwork would have prevented the error. In this case you will find seven "yes" answers to question 4 on the checklist.

Finally, as part of the retrospective analysis, a check of rater pair reliability was conducted using 16 cases. Two different p-n pairs each independently rated the 16 cases using the teamwork failure checklist. The results demonstrated good instrument reliability. There was a strong correspondence between the pairs with respect to total teamwork failure count ($r = +.85$, $p < .001$). Correspondence of judgments between the pairs for the global impact question (the three-level *Prevent/Mitigate/No Impact* scale) was good ($\tau_b = +.61$, $p = .006$).

Use of Teamwork Failure Assessments

The teamwork failure checklist can be used in a number of ways. It can help explain how an incident occurred and provide talking points for meeting with an upset family. Meeting in an honest, open fashion may help diffuse the anger and frustration and may actually reduce the risk of litigation. It can also allow periodic checks by management on the quality of the teamwork being provided. Reviewing a case's failures in various team dimensions provides management with a sense of where the problems lie. For example, a manager might discover that while the team structures are in place and the climate is supportive, the staff still demonstrate weak team communication habits. This finding would alert the clinical leaders as to where they need to focus teamwork sustainment training.

The checklist can also be used to assess and prepare cases for mortality and morbidity (M&M) conference presentations to the staff. It can also serve as the teamwork subanalysis in a root cause analysis conducted in response to a sentinel event. Recall that the Joint Commission guidance on sentinel events has identified weak teamwork as one of the Achilles heels in the health care system that is in need of repair.[46] Moreover, if multiple claims files exist, analysis of a set of checklists completed for five or ten other incidents would help an organization confirm the presence of teamwork failure trends that might be discovered in an RCA. Such trend data would reassure leadership that the action plan they had proposed in response to the sentinel event is on a sound footing. These potential uses of the teamwork failure checklist findings are described in more detail in table 9-3.

Because the reviewing of incidents almost always introduces legal concerns, any consideration of a review action should begin with a meeting with the risk manager. The risk manager must be involved in establishing rules for the control of the documents and any interactions with staff. The fact files needed to assess the teamwork performance must be handled with care so that legal privileges of the organization are not damaged.[47,48] In order to control legal risks, the risk manager should also be involved in any decisions regarding the release and use of the information.[49]

The p-n pair involved in incident review should be briefed by the risk manager on restrictions and protocols for accessing and using the claim fact files. Reviewers may be asked to sign nondisclosure agreements in order to gain access to files. Likewise, reviewers must adhere to any rules established regarding the distribution and protection of any notes and documents created.

Organizations must act aggressively to learn lessons and improve the care system, but they must do so in ways that avoid unreasonable

Table 9-3. Potential Uses of Teamwork Failure Checklist Findings

Use ID#	Use of Teamwork Failure Checklist Findings	Findings Derived from	Value of Findings to Organization/ Health Care Community	Risk Management Considerations in Use of Findings
1	Identify incident talking points for meeting with patient and family to explain incident.	Single case in own organization	Acknowledgment of a simple human failing may help diffuse anger and avoid litigation action; many patients and families are most concerned that the problem not happen again.	Consider establishing nondisclosure agreements with parties involved; consider access to and distribution of any acknowledgments with senior management and organization attorneys before meeting.
2	Limited in-house management review of teamwork weaknesses	Single case in own organization	• Flag possible teamwork problem areas and alert management to the possible need for training and management actions; may trigger training requirement or need for further trend analysis • Feedback to teamwork sustainment training efforts to improve performance	Restrict access to such a review; only show to senior management and managers directly involved in creating and implementing practical solutions; coordinate with risk manager to determine if a more in-depth analysis is appropriate and possible given the claim files available.
3	Case for morbidity/ mortality review: example of teamwork failure with serious consequences	Single case in own organization	Educate caregivers on specific teamwork failures that occurred and discuss important teamwork follow-through in future care management.	Provided to both physician and nursing staff as a normal part of the peer review process; parties appropriately cautioned not to discuss after M&M meeting has adjourned.
4	Root cause analysis (RCA) for a sentinel event: teamwork subanalysis	Single case in own organization	Addresses teamwork failures that contributed to the sentinel event and generates potential inputs to action plan	Carefully consider access to, and distribution of, any such analysis; only reveal results to senior management unless otherwise authorized.

266

Table 9-3. (Continued)

Use ID#	Use of Teamwork Failure Checklist Findings	Findings Derived from	Value of Findings to Organization/ Health Care Community	Risk Management Considerations in Use of Findings
5	In-house trend analysis to identify recurring teamwork problems unique to the organization	Multiple cases from own organization	Flag recurring teamwork problems and risks that exist in your own particular organization.	Restrict distribution of findings to senior management; reports that contain only statements of the problem should have a very limited distribution; reports that state problems and planned solutions may be more widely distributed.
6	Corroborate RCA findings regarding teamwork.	Multiple cases from own organization	Check that teamwork failures that have been identified in the RCA action plan are true recurring problems.	Attach as additional analysis action supporting the RCA; restrict access to those individuals authorized to see the RCA.
7	Research common teamwork failures that regularly occur in many health care organizations.	Multiple cases from multiple organizations	• Pooled data from sentinel events and/or closed cases allow identification of common recurring teamwork failures associated with major errors and significant indemnity costs. (Reactive research) • Pooled data from recent risk cases can allow early identification of emerging types of clinical error and associated teamwork breakdowns before they develop into major litigation areas (proactive research).	Only release data to research efforts where (1) data from multiple organizations are pooled and (2) only aggregate results will be reported; de-identify any cases released; restrict access to individual cases to a very small set of researchers and their assistants. Have all parties with access to individual interviews and completed checklists sign nondisclosure agreements.

legal risks. The actions and reactions of risk managers to a request for access to case facts may vary dramatically from one hospital to another. Their willingness or reluctance to help will be driven by the attitudes of the organization's senior leaders and the legal risks that are imposed by the laws of the particular state. If the senior leaders are not proactive and committed to preventive measures, gaining access to case files will be difficult.

It is also imperative that the managers and researchers conducting these assessments coordinate closely with the risk managers on use of the information generated. Senior leaders must consider carefully what information is to be released, to whom, in what form, and when it will be released. Some suggestions regarding risk management issues are shown in the last column of table 9-3. Recognize that these suggestions may require adjustments based on the tort laws of the particular state in which the organization resides.

IMPLEMENTING A TEAMWORK SYSTEM

Implementation of the MedTeams teamwork system involves a significant climate change for most EDs (as well as other units). Only a sustained commitment from senior leaders will make it happen.[50] They must ensure a supportive ED climate, work to change attitudes, and ensure that caregivers get significant training and practice until the new teamwork behaviors become habits. Senior leaders must support and work closely with the line-level implementers who oversee the daily teamwork training and practice in the department.

Senior leaders who should be involved and the roles they should play are listed below:[51]

- The chief executive officer is responsible for promoting the project vision at executive leadership levels, including board of director presentations.
- The vice president of clinical services is responsible for ensuring that the strategic plan envisions teamwork implementation and makes fiscal accommodations to ensure that this occurs.
- The human resource director is responsible for ensuring integration of teamwork factors into performance review process.

- The department physician director is responsible for ensuring that the strategic plan is integrated into the physician practice plan.
- The department nurse director is responsible for ensuring the strategic plan has the fiscal/operational support necessary to initiate and sustain teamwork implementation.
- Department clinical leadership is responsible for ensuring staff accountability for daily implementation of the teamwork system.

The basic types of support actions these senior leaders need to take are shown in figure 9-8. The particular attitudes and beliefs that must be encouraged for effective teamwork to emerge were discussed at the beginning of this chapter.

Figure 9-8.   Senior Leader Actions Necessary to Support Teamwork Implementation

1. Endorse the teamwork implementation initiative to board members, management, and staff as an important contributor to the control of clinical errors.
2. Select a strong physician-nurse pair (p-n pair) to lead implementation and send them to a teamwork training course.
3. Ensure that core care delivery teams (composed of physicians, nurses, and technicians) are established as part of the unit's standard daily work structure.
4. Revise policies to include procedures and protocols related to teamwork.
5. Include teamwork performance criteria in the personnel evaluation system.
6. Meet with the p-n pair on a regular basis to understand implementation difficulties and discuss possible solutions.
7. Include adequate implementation planning time in p-n pair work schedule.
8. Encourage staff to serve as program facilitators to aid implementation through support to the p-n pair.
9. Make a brief statement of organizational commitment to teamwork at the beginning of each training class.
10. Provide visible support and encouragement to the implementation leaders in the presence of the staff.
11. Hold teamwork implementation progress reviews.
12. Include teamwork failure analyses in root cause analyses of sentinel events.
13. Develop a sustainment strategy, including a plan for the replacement of teamwork implementation leaders as they move on.

A simplified conceptualization of the teamwork implementation process is shown in figure 9-9. While senior leadership commitment and support (shown at the top left) is clearly the driving force in implementation success, the sound execution of the four operational actions (shown in the middle) is the practical key to successful implementation. Action 1, selection and development of a physician-nurse pair, defines who will provide teamwork training for the staff and lead/facilitate the daily actions involved in implementation. This must be a seasoned physician-nurse pair that has the respect of the ED staff. They must have respect for each other and work well together. They may or may not be managers in the department but they must have the respect and support of the managers and senior leaders. This support must be provided as both protected time for planning/teaching/implementation/ evaluation and time for coordination with ED leadership to address the broad range of implementation issues that arise.

Use of a p-n pair in the teamwork implementation process is important because a critical part of the initiative is improving communication and coordination between physicians and nurses. These two individuals will come with their respective professional community's view of the ED and how it works. This pairing also symbolically demonstrates the core team structure on which the teamwork system is built. Ultimately, however, success will rest on the ability of the p-n pair to coordinate with each other, effectively communicate with the staff, and solve problems. They must be able to do the following:

- Lead actions that revise staff structure and create core teams
- Adjust management procedures to ensure maintenance of team structures over shift changes
- Establish schedules for staff teamwork training
- Deliver training to staff
- Determine fiscal support requirements
- Acquire and distribute implementation support materials (for example, core team identification devices such as scrubs, armbands, badges, training materials, and so on)
- Oversee team system start-up on the appointed day
- Establish teamwork coaching procedures and protocols to ensure that proper teamwork skills and habits are formed based on daily feedback

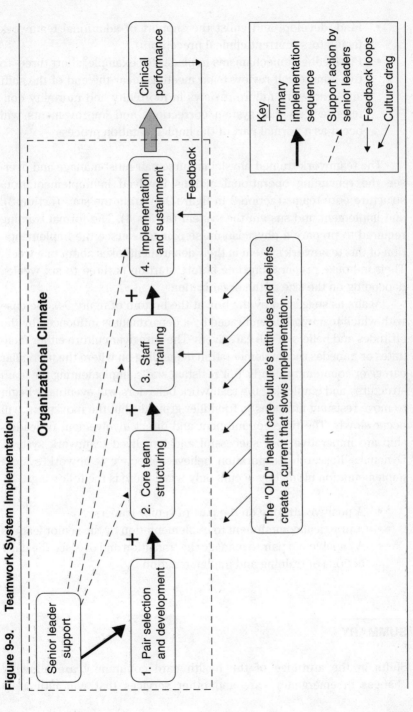

Figure 9-9.   Teamwork System Implementation

Organizational Climate

Senior leader support

1. Pair selection and development

2. Core team structuring

3. Staff training

4. Implementation and sustainment

Clinical performance

Feedback

+   +   +

The "OLD" health care culture's attitudes and beliefs create a current that slows implementation.

Key

Primary implementation sequence

Support action by senior leaders

Feedback loops

Culture drag

- Find, develop, and enlist the support of additional teamwork facilitators (current clinical preceptors)
- Put feedback mechanisms in place (for example, short three- to five-minute self-review team meetings near the end of the shift and teamwork failure reviews in morbidity and mortality conferences) so that system corrections and improvements will occur as a normal part of the implementation process

The teamwork-trained physician-nurse pair must manage and oversee the remaining operational actions involved in implementation: structure core teams (action 2 in figure 9-9), train the staff (action 3), and implement and sustain the system (action 4). The formal training required to prepare a physician-nurse pair to oversee the implementation of this teamwork system in their department takes about one week. Their in-house preparation time before start-up is three to six weeks, depending on the size of the organization.

Again, as suggested by the box at the bottom of figure 9-9, the ease with which teamwork is embraced by a department is influenced by the attitudes and beliefs of the caregivers. The caregiver culture either facilitates or impedes the implementation depending on where the particular caregiver community stands. For resistant staffs, implementing the team structures and employing the teamwork behaviors will eventually begin to move resistant attitudes to friendlier ground—but the movement will occur slowly. The time commitment and direct involvement of leadership are imperative to a successful and long-lived teamwork system. Dynamics Research Corporation believes effective teamwork system implementation ultimately occurs only when there is the following:

- A positive attitude on the part of senior leaders
- A practical commitment to implementation by the senior leaders
- A capable p-n pair to manage the transition and oversee the daily actions of training and implementation

SUMMARY

Shifts in the attitudes of the health care community are allowing changes in emergency care and other services that will ultimately improve care delivery and reduce the error rates associated with care. Movement toward these newer attitudes and beliefs significantly improves the opportunities for teamwork system implementation. In particular, changes in caregiver beliefs and attitudes regarding personal fallibility, work approach, care system complexity, primary source of clinical error, peer checks of one's actions, and caregiver skills required will make teamwork implementation easier.

Finally, existing research suggests that improved teamwork can have a profound impact on ED patient care.[52] The teamwork concepts discussed here, the teamwork system that is emerging, and the teamwork failure checklist tool for assessing teamwork performance in incidents are devices that will improve the teamwork component of health care. The ultimate key to implementation lies in the willingness of the organization's senior leaders to commit to the initiative. With senior leadership commitment and a little patience and perseverance, caregivers will learn coordination skills and communication habits that will enable them to better integrate their clinical actions and implement a team-based, patient-focused cultural change. And, at least as important, caregivers will learn to more openly accept help from others to avoid the inevitable errors that are part of being human.

ACKNOWLEDGMENTS*

We are deeply indebted to the vision of Dr. Dennis Leedom of the Army Research Laboratory, who initiated this project and his outstanding successor, Mr. Mike Golden of the Army Research Laboratory, who has chaperoned it through all phases. We also wish to thank the visionary leaders of the participating hospitals who recognized that improving teamwork was important even before the Joint Commission raised the visibility of the issue. But most important, we wish to thank the exceptional doctors and nurses they sent us, the members of the MedTeams Consortium,[53] for their dedication, diligence, insight, perseverance, sense of humor, and willingness to step into the breach to make this sea

*The MedTeams research reported in this chapter was supported by contract DAAL01-96-C-0091 from the Army Research Laboratory. The views, opinions, and findings expressed are those of the authors and should not be construed as an official position of the U.S. Department of Defense or its agencies.

change occur. We also owe a great debt to Roland Loranger, Joseph Melino, and Joan Flynn of Lifespan Risk Management for their willingness to educate us about incidents, claims, and the world of risk management. And finally we wish to thank Dr. Lucian Leape of the Harvard School of Public Health for his encouragement and support when we were just a small group initiating the project and for his long perseverance in surfacing and framing the problem of error in medicine.

References and Notes

1.   *American Heritage Dictionary*, 2d ed. (Boston: Houghton Mifflin Co., 1982).

2.   R. Helmreich. "Managing Human Error in Aviation," *Scientific American* 276, no. 5 (May 1997): 62–67.

3.   G. Grubb et al. "Effects of Crew Coordination Training and Evaluation Methods on AH-64 Attack Helicopter Battalion Crew Performance," working paper (Fort Rucker, AL: U.S. Army Research Institute, Aviation Research and Development Activity, 1993), pp. 14–17.

4.   D. Leedom and R. Simon. "Improving Team Coordination: A Case for Behavior-Based Training," *Military Psychology* 7, no. 2 (February 1995): 109–22.

5.   A. Gayman et al. "Implications of Crew Resource Management Training For Tank Crews," conference presentation, Interservice/Industry Training System and Education Conference, Orlando, FL (December 1996).

6.   Ibid.

7.   G. Grubb et al. "Effects of Crew Coordination Training," pp. 14–17.

8.   J. Reason and K. Mycielska. *Absent-Minded? The Psychology of Mental Lapses and Everyday Errors* (Englewood Cliffs, NJ: Prentice Hall, 1982).

9.   J. Reason. *Human Error* (New York: Cambridge University Press, 1990).

10. L. Koss. "Cervical (PAP) Smear: New Directions," *Cancer Supplement* 71, no. 4 (1993): 1406–12.

11. S. Bogner, ed. *Human Error in Medicine* (Hillsdale, NJ: Lawrence Erlbaum Associates, 1994).

12. L. Leape et al. "The Nature of Adverse Events in Hospitalized Patients: Results of the Harvard Medical Practice Study II," *NEJM* 324, no. 6 (1991): 377–84.

13. L. Leape. "Error in Medicine," *JAMA* 272, no. 23 (December 21, 1994): 1851–57.

14. L. L. Leape. "Errors in Health Care: Problems and Challenges," conference presentation, Examining Errors In Health Care: Developing a Prevention, Education, and Research Agenda, Rancho Mirage, CA (October 13, 1996).

15. E. Bartlett. "Physicians, Cognitive Errors, and Their Liability Consequences," *Journal of Healthcare Risk Management* 18, no. 4 (April 1998): 62–69.

16. P. Weiler et al. *A Measure of Malpractice: Medical Injury, Malpractice Litigation, & Patient Compensation* (Cambridge, MA: Harvard University Press, 1993).

17. L. Leape. "Error in Medicine," pp. 1851–57.

18. L. L. Leape, "Errors in Health Care: Problems and Challenges."

19. S. Bogner, ed. *Human Error in Medicine*.

20. R. Simon et al. *Full Scale Development of Emergency Team Coordination Course (ETCC) and Evaluation Measures* (Andover, MA: Dynamics Research Corporation, 1997), p. 20.

21. M. Chassin, R. Galvin, and National Roundtable on Health Care Quality. "The Urgent Need to Improve Health Care Quality," *JAMA* 280, no. 11 (September 16, 1998): 1000–1005.

22. D. Dorner. *The Logic of Failure: Recognizing and Avoiding Error in Complex Situations* (New York: Metropolitan Books, 1996).

23. J. Schmidt and G. P. Moore. "Management of Multiple Trauma," *Emergency Medicine Clinics of North America* 11, no. 1 (February 1993): 29–51.

24. Joint Commission on Accreditation of Healthcare Organizations. *Sentinel Events: Evaluating Cause and Planning Improvement* (Oakbrook Terrace, IL: Joint Commission, 1998).

25. L .S. Binder and D. M. Chapman. "Qualitative Research Methodologies in Emergency Medicine," *Acad Emerg Med* 2, no. 12 (December 1995): 1098–1102.

26. M. L. Millenson. *Demanding Medical Excellence: Doctors and Accountability in the Information Age* (Chicago: University of Chicago Press, 1997).

27. L. L. Leape, "Error in Medicine," pp. 1851–57.

28. Y. Xiao et al. and the LOTAS Group. "Task Complexity in Emergency Medical Care and Its Implications for Team Coordination," *Human Factors* 38, no. 4 (April 1996): 636–45.

29. M. Chassin, R. Galvin, and National Roundtable on Health Care Quality, "The Urgent Need to Improve Health Care Quality," pp. 1000–1005.

30. C. Vincent, S. Taylor-Adams, and N. Stanhope. "Framework for Analyzing Risk and Safety in Clinical Medicine." *BMJ* 316, no. 7138 (April 11, 1998): 1154–57.

31. Joint Commission on Accreditation of Healthcare Organizations. *Sentinel Events.*

32. L. Leape et al. "The Nature of Adverse Events in Hospitalized Patients," pp. 377–84.

33. L. Leape. "Error in Medicine," pp. 1851–57.

34. D. Gaba. "Human Error in Dynamic Medical Domains," in S. Bogner, ed., *Human Error in Medicine* (Hillsdale, NJ: Lawrence Erlbaum Associates, 1994).

35. R. Simon et al. *Full Scale Development of Emergency Team Coordination Course*, p. 16.

36. Ibid.

37. R. Simon et al. "Reducing Errors in Emergency Medicine Through Team Performance: The MedTeams Project," conference presentation, in the Proceedings of Enhancing Patient Safety and Reducing Errors in Healthcare, Rancho Mirage, CA (November 8–10, 1998).

38. D. Risser et al. and MedTeams Consortium, "The Potential for Improved Teamwork to Reduce Medical Errors in the ED," *Annals of Emergency Medicine* (in press).

39. R. Simon et al. "Reducing Errors."

40. D. Risser et al. and MedTeams Consortium, "The Potential for Improved Teamwork."

41. For more information about the MedTeams Project, visit the project Web site at: http://teams.drc.com.

42. M. Endsley. "Toward a Theory of Situation Awareness in Dynamic Systems," *Human Factors* 37, no. 1 (March 1995): 32–64.

43. A subproject within the MedTeams Project is exploring the use of ultra-light-weight, portable communication devices (with controllable channels) to enable team members to speak to each other at a distance. This capability may significantly enhance the ability of the team to communicate essential information without the members needing to convene at a single physical point. This could significantly enhance the ability of the team to coordinate and maintain situation awareness.

44. A. Locke et al. *Instructor Guide for Emergency Team Coordination Course (ETCC)* (Andover, MA: Dynamics Research Corporation, 1997). pp. 1–9.

45. Joint Commission on Accreditation of Healthcare Organizations. *Sentinel Events.*

46. Ibid., p. 129.

47. E. Barton. "Claims and Litigation Management," in R. Carroll, ed., *Risk Management Handbook for Healthcare Organizations*, 2d ed (Chicago: American Hospital Publishing, Inc., 1997).

48. K. Davis and J. McConnell. "Data Management," in R. Carroll, ed., *Risk Management Handbook for Healthcare Organizations.*

49. M. Sassano and J. Dronsfeld. "Securing Risk Management Information From Discovery," in G. Henry, ed., *Emergency Medicine Risk Management: A Comprehensive Review* (Dallas: American College of Emergency Physicians, 1991), pp. 201–5.

50. K. Phillips. *The Power of Health Care Teams: Strategies for Success* (Oakbrook Terrace, IL: Joint Commission, 1997), p. 105.

51. Recognize that while the official titles listed may change from one facility to another, the basic roles and responsibilities will exist for most institutions.

52. D. Risser et al. and MedTeams Consortium, "The Potential for Improved Teamwork."

53. Gary Adamowicz, BS; Steven L. Banks, DO; Scott Berns, MD, MPH, FAAP; MAJ Tammie Chang, RN, MSN, CEN; Capt. James Cleveland, RN; Capt. Robin Cody, RN, EMT-B, CEN; Teresa Czaplinski, RN, BSN; James Evangelista, RN, RPh, CEN; LTC Daniel Fitzpatrick, DO, MPH; Nancy Gates; Marjorie Geist, RN, MSN, MHA, PhD; Amy Guilfoil-Dumont, RN; Lori A. Hughes, RN, MS, CEN; Bruce Janiak, MD; Gregory D. Jay, MD, PhD, FACEP; Jorie Klein, RN; Vinette Langford, RN-CS, MSN, CEN; CPT Constance Lavieri-Reynolds, MD; Lt. Col. Thomas Lenz, MD; Ann Locke, RN-CS, MSN; Sandra McDonald, RN, BSN; CDR Timothy McGuirk, DO, FACEP; John C. Morey, PhD, CHFP; Todd Murray, MD; Dallas E. Peak, MD, FACEP; Shawna J. Perry, MD; LCDR James R. Pierce, RN, MSN, CEN; COL Matthew M. Rice, MD, JD, FACEP; Daniel Risser, PhD; Laura Rodgers, RN, MSN, CEN, CCRN, William D. Rose, MD, FACEP; Mary Salisbury, RN, MSN; Robert Simon, EdD, CPE; Harry Swiger, RN, BA; Carla G. Tolbert, MS, RN, CCRN, CEN; LTC Clyde Turner, DO, MPH; Robert L. Wears, MD, MS, FACEP; Kenneth A. Williams, MD, FACEP; Charlotte S. Yeh, MD, FACEP.

Index

Accident(s), 98
 issues surrounding health care,
  xxv–xxvi
 medical, xxvi–xxvii, xxviii, 119–31
 single-error, 6
 system behavior in, 110–13
Accident investigations, xxvi, 141
 active errors and latent system faults,
  141–42
 and anticipatory failure analysis in
  hospitals, 139–52
 hospital, 143–46
Accident trajectory, 113–14
Active errors, xxiii, 5
 in accident investigations, 141–42
 examples of, 5
Active failures, 110–11, 117, 118
 identifying, 125
Administrative data, 66–69
Administrative databases, 68–69
Adverse drug reactions, identifying in
  medical records, 70–71
Adverse events, 24–25
Aggregate data analysis, 45
American Academy of Pediatrics (AAP),
  212
American Medical Association, formation
  of National Patient Safety
  Foundation by, xxii
American Society of Anesthesiologists, 8
 Closed Claims Project of, 85
American Society of Hospital Pharmacists
  (ASHP), 212
Anesthesia, studies of critical incidents
  in, 85
Anesthesia Patient Safety Foundation,
  xxv
Anesthesiology, error management in, 200
Annenberg Conference on Examining
  Errors in Health Care, xxi

Anticipatory failure analysis, 146, 149–50
Asphyxia, xxviii
Autoimmune deficiencies, patients with,
  20
Automated drug dispensing, xxii
Automation, 224–27
 errors enabled by, 225–27
 value of, for root cause analysis,
  166–67

Benchmarking
 competitive, 80, 82–87
 internal, 79–80
 performance, 79–87
Bias, confirmation, 104
Billing data, 66
Billing database, 66–67
BRAVO, 177

CARA-FaultTree, 177
Case reviews, 18
Checklists, 9
Chemotherapy, improving safety in, 219
Chunking of information, 101–5
Clinical pathway, 205
Clinical practice guidelines, 205
Closed Claims Project of the American
  Society of Anesthesiologists, 85
Cognitive fixation, 104
Cognitive lock-up, 104
Communication, improving, in error man-
  agement strategies, 211
Competitive benchmarking, 80, 82–87
Complex system, 97
Comprehensive error reduction initiative,
  26
Computerized decision aids, xxvii, 9
Computerized physician ordering sys-
  tems, xxii
Confirmation bias, 104

Constraining functions, 209
Contributing causes, identifying, 125–26
Control charts, 77–79
    versus run charts, 79
Cross-monitoring failure, 239, 241

Data analysis
    aggregate, 45
    techniques in, 74–79
Data organization, improved, in root
        cause analysis (RCA) automa-
        tion, 156–57
Data point, 78
Decision Systems, Inc., 162
Defective barriers, xxii
Depression, patient under treatment for,
        20
Diagnosis codes, problems with use of,
        67
Disturbance-Effect-Barrier (DEB) analy-
        sis, 131, 150
    case study, 132–35
Drug reactions. *See also* Medication
        errors
    identifying adverse, in medical
        records, 70–71
Dynamics Research Corporation, 237,
        239, 258, 272

E-codes, 66–67
Emergency care, teamwork challenges in,
        238–41
Environment, adjusting, 210–11
Equipment problems, 220, 222–24
Error(s). *See also* Medication errors
    active, xxiii, 5, 141–42
    containment of, 17
        identifying and implementing
            action plans, 134–35
    eliminating consequences of, 203
    elimination of, 202
    enabled by automation, 225–27
    human, xxi, 4–5
    latent, xxii
    measurement of, xxiii
    mitigating effects of, 191–92
    number of potentially preventable
        medical, 3
    prevention of, xxi, xxii
    safety-critical, 7

Error management, 17, 201–17
    adjusting environment in, 210–11
    adjusting work schedules in, 210
    constraints in, 209
    decreasing reliance on vigilance in,
        211–14
    designing for, 209–10
    forcing functions in, 209
    improving communication in, 211
    improving information access in,
        208–9
    multiple work system improvements
        in, 216–17
    personal approach to, 200
    providing adequate safety training in,
        215
    purpose of performance measure-
        ments in, 18
    reliance on memory in, 204–7
    role of Man-Technique-Organization
        (MTO) analysis in, 131–35
    simplifying process/reducing hand-
        offs in, 203–4
    staffing in, 215–16
    standardizing, 207–8
Error proofing, 7–10
Error reduction, 17
    achieving goals, 18
    in health care, xxv
    strategies in, 8–9
    structured teamwork system in,
        235–74
    system redesign in, 8
    work system improvements in,
        199–228
Event mapping, 124–25

Failure mode, 193
Failure Mode and Effect Analysis
        (FMEA), 149, 188–89
Failure Modes, Effects, and Criticality
        Analysis (FMECA), 159
Falls, 20
FaultTree+, 177
Fault Tree Analysis (FTA), 149–50, 189
Faulty systems, relationship between
        human errors and, 4–5
Flawed safety barrier, 115
FMEA (Failure Mode and Effect
        Analysis), 149

FMECA (Failure Modes, Effects, and Criticality Analysis), 159
Food and Drug Administration (FDA) MedWatch Program, 25
Forcing functions, 209
FTA (Fault Tree Analysis), 149–50, 189

General risk-related performance measures, 27–30
Good root cause analysis, goal of, 179

HACCP (Hazard Analysis and Critical Control Point), 149
Hand-offs, reducing number of, 9, 10
Harvard Medical Practice, 20
Harvard Medical System, 86
Hazop (Hazard and Operability Study), 149
Health care
    issues surrounding accidents in, xxv–xxvi
    medical management of, 188–95
        determining treatment, 189–92
        diagnosis, 188–89
        follow-up, 194–95
        implementing treatment, 192–94
    performance measures for, 17–18
    proactively error-proofing, 179–97
Health care system failure, 109
High-risk patient groups, 19–20
High-risk processes, 20–22, 151
    definition of, 19
    measuring performance of, 17–87
    monitoring, 18–22
Hospitals
    accident investigations in, 139–52, 143–46
    anticipatory failure analysis in, 139–52
    patient injury in, 20
    patient safety improvement structure in, 150–51
Human errors
    causes of, xxi
    relationship between faulty systems and, 4–5
Human factors engineering, 8, 210
Human fallibility, 7
Humans as problem solvers, 99–108
Human-system interface, 109–19
Human-system misfits, 97

Identification bands
    importance of, 6
    outdated equipment in producing, 6
Incident reports, 38–66
    gross underreporting of medication errors through, 74, 76
    quantity and quality of, 40
Incidents, identifying teamwork failures in, 253–68
Information
    chunking of, 101–5
    improving access to, 9–10, 208–9
Inspection logs, 222
Institute for Healthcare Improvement (IHI), 218
    National Collaborative on Reducing Adverse Drug Events and Medical Errors, 41
Institute for Safe Medication Practices (ISMP), xxv, 85–86, 205, 212–13
Internal benchmarking, 79–80
International Classification of Diseases, Ninth Revision, Clinical Modification (ICD-9-CM), 66–67
ISO 9000 international standard for quality management, 111
ISO 9001 standard for quality assurance, 111

JBF Associates, Inc., 162
Joint Commission on Accreditation of Healthcare Organizations (JCAHO), xxii, xxv
    and accident investigation, 139
    accreditation standards, 22, 31, 74
    and process changes, 216
    and root cause analysis, 155, 165
    and sentinel events, 20, 25, 86, 253

Knowledge-based problem solving, 106, 107–8

Latent errors, xxii
Latent failures, 110–11, 112, 115, 117–18, 119
    identifying ineffective, 126, 128, 130
Latent system faults, 5–6
    in accident investigations, 141–42
Long-term memory, 99

Malpractice claims
    analysis of data, 19
    information in, 66
Man-Technique-Organization (MTO)
        analysis, 98–99, 120–21, 121–30
    acting on results, 130–31
    role of, in error management, 131–35
    steps of, 120
    training and support of teams in, 121
Measurement data, collecting, 31–32
Medical accidents, xxvi–xxvii, xxviii
    framework for investigating, 119–31
Medical Device Amendments (1992), 85
Medical errors, number of potentially
        preventable, 3
Medical management of health care
        process, 188–95
    determining treatment, 189–92
    diagnosis, 188–89
    follow-up, 194–95
    implementing treatment, 192–94
Medical mistakes
    costs associated with, xxviii
    human side of, 97–137
Medical records, 69–72
    cost of retrospective review of, 69–70
    identifying adverse drug reactions in,
        70–71
    ownership of, xxviii
Medication errors, xxi–xxii, xxviii. *See
        also* Drug reactions; Error(s)
    definition of, 24, 41
    gross underreporting of, through inci-
        dent reports, 74, 76
    protecting against, 217–20
    tips for reducing, in physician's office,
        221–22
Medication flow sheet, 222
Medication use
    as high-risk activity, 20–22
    measuring performance of, 21–22
MedTeams Project, 241, 242
    activities in, 247, 250, 252–53
    definition and composition, 242
    implementation of teamwork system,
        268–72
    responsibilities in, 242, 244
    teamwork dimensions and behaviors
        in, 244, 246–47
Memory
    long-term, 99

    reducing reliance on, 9
    in error management strategies,
        204–7
    working, 100
Minimum Data Set (MDS), 68
Mistakes
    definition of, 4
    medical, xxviii, 97–137
    reasons for, 4–7

NASA's Aviation Safety Reporting System
    (ASRS), 84–85
National Center for Missing and
    Exploited Children, 213
National Collaborative on Reducing
    Adverse Drug Events and Med-
    ical Errors, 41
National Coordinating Council for Med-
    ication Error Reporting and
    Prevention (NCC MERP), 50
National Patient Safety Foundation, xxv
    formation of, xxii
National Practitioner Data Bank, 83–84
Near-miss behavior, identification of pat-
    terns of, 23
Near-miss events, xxvi–xxvii, xxviii
New York Patient Occurrence Reporting
    and Tracking System
    (NYPORTS), 84

Occurrence report, 7
"One cell-one cause," 125
Organization, 97
Outcome and Assessment Information
    Set (OASIS), 68–69
Outcome measures, 24, 25
Outcome screens, 69
Outliers, xxiii

Patient care logs, 72
Patient Encounter Worksheet, 69
Patient identification, 6
Patient records. *See* Medical records
Patient safety, xxi, xxvi
    improving, xxvii
    proactive initiatives, xxvii
    problems as predictor of, 21
    purpose of performance measures, 23
Patient surveys, 72
Pediatric Perioperative Cardiac Arrest
    Registry (POCA), 85

Performance measurements, 23–31
  analysis of, 72–87
  general risk-related, 27–30
  for high-risk processes, 17–87
  outcome, 25
  process, 24–25
  purpose of, in error management, 18
  safety-critical tasks, 26, 31
  uses of, 23
Performance shaping factors, 108
PHA-Pro, 177
Physician order sheet, 205
Point-of-care documentation systems, 69
Pressure ulcers, 20
PROACT, 177
Proactive analysis, 158–59
Proactive error-proofing for health care
    processes, 179–97
Proactive patient safety initiatives, xxvii
Proactive risk-reduction activities, check-
    list for, 196
Problem solving
  humans in, 99–108
  knowledge-based, 106, 107–8
  rule-based, 106, 107
  skill-based, 106
  system factors influencing, 108
Problem space, 108
Procedure codes, problems with use of,
    67
Processes
  anatomy and physiology of, 180–81
  definition of, 180–81
  failure of, 181–84
  methods of error-proofing, 7–10
  reasons for failure of, 184–87
    complexity, 185
    hierarchical culture, 187
    human intervention, 186–87
    inconsistency, 185–86
    tight coupling, 186
    tight time constraints, 187
    variable input, 184–85
  simplifying, in error management
    strategies, 203–4
Process measures, 23–25
Process redesign in reducing error occur-
    rence, 202–3
Process reliability, improving, 131
Process variance, 24
Prospective systems analysis, xxiii

Protocols, 9
Psychological factors, 7

Quality improvement teams, xxii
Quality management activities, 6

Reactive analysis, 158–59
REASON, 177
Redundancy, 191
Reliability Center, Inc., 163
Reliance, decreasing, on vigilance, 211–14
Retrospective case-by-case review, 18
Retrospective record review, cost of,
    69–70
Risk Management Incident Collaborative,
    86
Risk-related performance measures
  compiling, 73–74
  reporting inconsistencies in, 76
Root cause analysis (RCA), xxvi–xxvii,
    111, 139–41, 179
  automating, 155–64
    advantages of, 156–58
    desirable features, 158–62
  definition of, 155
  matching features with products,
    175–77
  in sentinel event occurrence, 150–51
  software facilitation of, 165–77
  value of automation, 166–67
Root cause analysis software
  choices in, 162–63
  evaluation criteria, 167–75
    confidentiality, 174
    cost, 175
    database functionality, 173–74
    data entry, 169–70
    ease of use, 169
    graphics, 173
    hierarchical security, 175
    LAN capabilities/data integration,
      174
    noncontributing factors, 171
    operational logic flow, 171–72
    output, 172–73
    philosophy, 168–69
    search function, 174
    terminology, 170
    tools, 171
    training capacity, 172
    validity, 170–71
    Windows compliant, 169

Rule-based problem solving, 106, 107
Run charts, 76–77
    versus control charts, 79

Safe Medical Devices Act (1990), 85
Safety barriers, 112–13
    flawed, 115
    identifying ineffective, 126, 128, 130
Safety-critical errors, 7
Safety-critical features in equipment,
        224–25
Safety-critical patient care activities,
        identifying, xxvi
Safety-critical tasks
    definition of, 26
    measuring, 26, 31
Safety-related data, reporting inconsisten-
        cies in, 74, 76
Safety-related structural components,
        measures of, 24
Safety training, providing adequate, 215
SAPHIRE, 177
Schema, 103
Schematas, 101
Sentinel events, xxiii, 25, 98, 146, 179
    causes of, xxvii
    root cause analysis requirement for
        occurrence, 150–51
Single-error accidents, 6
Situational factors, xxii, 111–12, 115–17,
        118–19
    identifying, 125–26
Skill-based problem solving, 106
Software facilitation of root cause analy-
        sis, 165–77
Special computerized databases, 72
Staffing, inadequacy of, 5
Staff surveys, 72
Standardizing in error management
        strategies, 207–8
System behavior in accidents, 110–13
System factors, influencing problem
        solving, 108

System failure, 109
System Improvements, Inc., 163
System redesign, importance of, as error
        reduction strategy, 8
Systems approach, intellectual basis for,
        xxii–xxiii

TapRooT, 177
Tasks, standardizing, 9, 10
Team training, xxiii
Teamwork
    challenges in emergency care, 238–41
    definition of, 235
    implementing system, 268–72
    structured, in reducing clinical errors,
        235–74
    tactics for enhancing, xxvii–xxviii
Teamwork Behavior Matrix, 247
Teamwork check cycle, 250, 252
Teamwork Failure Checklist, 237–38
Teamwork failures
    identifying, in incidents, 253–68
    use of assessments, 264–65, 268
Teamwork implementation process, 270

Unlucky circumstances, 111–12
Unnecessary surgery incidents, 3–4
Untoward event, 98

Veterans Health Administration (VHA),
        xxv, 86–87
Vigilance, decreasing, reliance on, 211–14

"What if" question, xxiii
Working memory, 100
Work schedules, adjusting, 210
Work system improvements
    need for multiple, 216–17
    reducing errors through, 199–228
"Worst-case" analysis, 189